Autism: The

Recovering the Self through Heilkunst

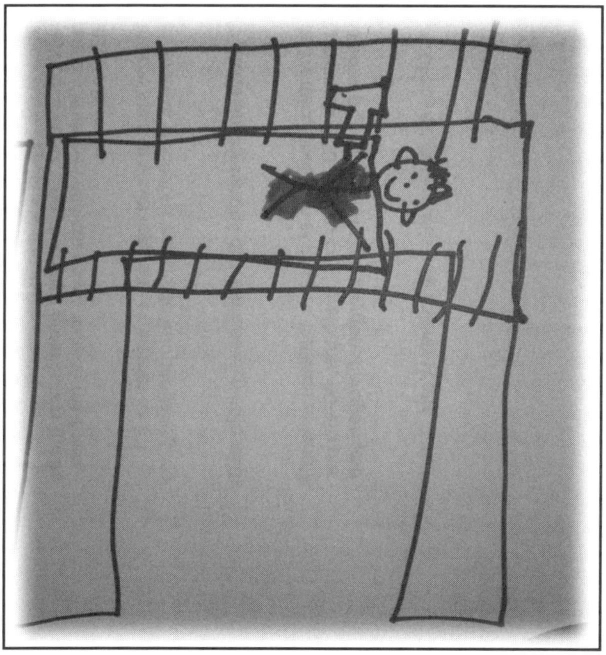

Rudi Verspoor, FHCH, HD(RHom.), DMH
Patty Smith, FHCH, HD(RHom.), DMH

Autism: The Journey Back - Recovering the Self
Through Heilkunst

www.homeopathy.com
www.heilkunst.com

ISBN 0-9685166-9-6

Cover design by Eric Verspoor

Cover art by Sebastien

Description:

The doctor hurt the boy with the needle:

This is a drawing my son, Sebastien, produced spontaneously and has expressed as:

"The doctor hurt the boy with the needle."

You will note the boy is in a crib -- his drawing resembles his own crib with the solid headboard, which he hasn't seen for at least four years. As well, he hasn't been exposed to inoculations since his 18 month shots. Sebastien explained several times that he was the boy on the picture and showed precisely where he was inoculated. Note the syringe.

My only question is whether he is referring to his 18-month shot or his 12-month shot. Historically we see his 12-month shot as the time when his health dipped. There was no prompting whatsoever, and Sebastien's drawing was absolutely spontaneous.

His drawing raise all kinds of questions:

1) Sebastien remembers that his inoculation hurt him badly; this is especially significant as we just completed the remedies for his 18-month DPT remedies and are about to engage in the remedies for his 12-month MMR shot. I'm still unsure which one he is referring to in his drawing, as his reaction to the MMR shots was manifold worse than his reaction to the DPT shots.

If he is referring to his 18-month shot, then I can only speculate that the healing reaction to his 12-month shots will be immensely painful to all of us.

2) He is able to get a temporal fix on the time at which he became ill; this is formidable.

3) He remembers the arm in which he was inoculated.

4) This drawing has been recurrent over the past three days. He has made dozens of them and he keeps repeating, “The doctor hurt the boy with the needle.” I'm assuming that this is a critical part of the healing process and my approach is to let him be with that.

5) In the past he has focussed on drawing toilets. Today he has been drawing both toilets and himself in the crib. I'm speculating that the toilets are a representation of his fear -- I remember toilet training him was hell as he was deathly scared of toilets."

Autism: The Journey Back

"Maria previously had to set goals with her teacher, mostly about managing her emotions, and one of the main ones was for her to become more self-regulating. She was having one or two meltdowns a day, and was hard for the teacher to manage.

After her first set of Heilkunst remedies the three of us had a parent-teacher interview, and when the teacher asked her how she was doing and how she would renew her goals, Maria said she hadn't needed to use her coping tactics because she didn't have reason to. The teacher thought for a moment and realized she was right!

And though she is usually a loner at lunch, her teacher looked up from her desk one afternoon to hear two girls busily chatting away, the conversation going back and forth and laughing their heads off. The teacher said she was shocked to see that one of the girls was Maria!"

Dedication

This book would not have been written without the help of so many others. We would first like to thank our children (all five), who taught us many things about life and love, and the challenges of raising kids in a modern world – they showed us the best and the most challenging aspects of growing up, and also how to tap into the incredible potential for creativity that they represent. Without them we would not have the insight into childhood behavioral problems that we now have and how they can be converted from dross to gold through a modern form of alchemy, energetic medicine.

We would next like to thank the many parents and children who have trusted us enough to come for treatment to show that it works, consistently and effectively, and to challenge us to go further each time, just when we might become complacent. When we might have lost some hope, they persisted and encouraged us with their trust to continue through our sometimes difficult, sometimes humbling, yet always stimulating and exciting education about the autistic condition.

We'd also like to thank all of our students who, at various stages, came to learn, but also to challenge any preconceptions or confusion of mind, and to encourage us to understand better so that we might explain better. If this is to benefit many, it will be because of those others who practice Heilkunst and apply its principles of scientific medicine.

Our sincere thanks also to the staff of the Hahnemann Center, its Clinic and College, who have supported all of these efforts and worked tirelessly in the background to make it all possible.

And finally, our thanks to those dedicated individuals who took the time to thoroughly proof our work, and to offer constructive advice—Venetia Diamond and Caroline Ross. Any errors or omissions remain the sole responsibility of the authors.

Preview

We face a modern plague of biblical proportions and it is affecting mainly our children. An increasing number are born into this world, but do not seem to be fully of this world – they appear to live in a world of their own making, often full of fear and confusion. These children have difficulty communicating, interacting and behaving "normally." It's as if a modern Pied Piper has beguiled them and taken them away to a strange land behind a glass wall, which we cannot, as parents, friends, educators and practitioners, seem to penetrate. We now have an ever lengthening alphabet soup of letters and terms to describe these "lost" children – ADHD, ADD, PDD, OCD, ODD – children who are all on what has been termed the "autistic spectrum."

This book is about all those children who find themselves on that spectrum and to their parents and family. Its main intent is to set out an effective approach to bring these children back into the world of ordinary consciousness, to help them to reclaim their true self. Our main contention is that autism is not a disease as such, but an attempt of the human organism to hold a precarious balance in the face of various underlying blockages, shocks and traumas. The key to defeating autism is to remove these underlying causes so that the child no longer needs the various symptoms of the autistic condition to deal with the outside world.

The essence of the autistic condition is a loss of the self through the unprecedented assault on each child from the moment of conception to age 3, when the self emerges, as a conscious entity in each child. It is a descent into a realm full of anxiety, fear, confusion, and unpredictability, the natural, primitive world of the sub-conscious that the 19th Century psychologist, William James, called "bloomin', buzzin' confusion." Without a clear sense of self, we lose the ability to distinguish between what is going on outside and inside, between dream consciousness and waking reality.

At the same time, it is not only the shocks and traumas that are responsible. There must also be a certain weakness inherent in the unique make-up of each child that allows these assaults to result in an autistic condition. For example, not all children vaccinated or exposed to thimerosal or to birth traumas become autistic. The level of heavy metals in autistic children is not found in others in their family or immediate environment. Indeed, we have come across the case of twins, one of whom was diagnosed autistic, the other not. In essence, the autistic condition has multiple causes, many typical, but the combination is unique to that child.

At the same time, these children are found to have various chemical, hormonal and nutritional imbalances, not to mention various allergic reactions to certain foods. It is important to address these concerns, and to provide the best possible foundation for health, but also to recognize that many of these imbalances are themselves caused by the various shocks and traumas and the inherent weaknesses they trigger. To simply chelate or detoxify, or to provide various other therapies only addresses the symptoms without addressing the underlying causes.

Heilkunst is a comprehensive, integrated system of Western medicine based on the principles of natural law regarding the removal of disease (cure) and the restoration of balance in our functioning (healing). The essence of Heilkunst, which encompasses regimen as well as medicine proper, is not the remedy, but the process. Most cases of autism are complex in nature. The initial inherited weaknesses, various birth shocks, vaccinations, drugs and other traumas to the developing self in the first few years of life produce secondary effects, such as digestive problems, weak immune systems, aberrant behavior, sleep disorders, fungal overgrowth, heavy metal toxicity, food sensitivities and chemical reactions, which also need to be addressed before the energetic medicines can properly work. The solution lies in a systematic, logical, causally-grounded process that can address each of these factors within a clear context so that the practitioner does not get lost in the swamp of symptoms, or simply put out fires, rather than dealing with what is *setting* these "fires."

A part of this book is also an attempt to understand the emergence of autistic behavior in so many children in what amounts to a cultural phenomenon. In more traditional societies, the meaning of illness is part of the process of cure and healing. In our empirical and materially-oriented world, we tend to focus on the simple elimination of a presumed disease or condition. However, the real causes can only emerge through a deeper understanding of a given condition. In a profound spiritual sense illness is part of the human condition and part of a higher design. It is in the struggle against disease and illness that we can ultimately find ourselves. In our struggle with this profound disturbance of childhood in our time, we are forced to confront the meaning of many aspects of our culture, where it is headed and what our role is in its evolution. Our children become very much our teachers. The challenge is to understand what they are teaching us. What is offered here is only a beginning.

"Instead of questions for you I have something to tell you. We've noticed that Grace is doing much, much better. Her overall demeanor has improved so much! She seems to be coming out of her shell, she's more playful, she imitates us more, she wants to interact with us more and make arm gestures when we sing songs to her (she never did that before), and sometimes she'll even try to imitate a small sound that we make. We are unbelievably happy with just this improvement.

I realized how much she had improved when Grace and I went to meet her new Speech Language Pathologist who just happens to be on the Autism Team in our city. Grace did about 95% of what they asked of her (except speech). They told me they're seeing such great things (not autism per se) but they did confirm that she has a couple of things that are on the spectrum. That's when I realized that it did not matter what they "label" her because homeopathy and Heilkunst will tear down each barrier until she can be who she is supposed to be. The SLP thought that perhaps she has apraxia... but not complete apraxia. Well it doesn't matter what she has.

When Grace had her Fair Start Screening in October 2004 (prior to me contacting you) she did not do most of what the lady asked of her... apparently she scored 1/12. She wasn't having a great day, mind you. In fact she barely looked at her, she barely looked at us and she did not even want to sit on my or her dad's lap. She didn't point to her body parts when asked even though she knew them. Wow, she has improved so much since then and we are so grateful.

We know we still have a long way to go but just seeing some improvement is by far worth the wait!"

Table of Contents

1| Introduction

Autism, by dictionary definition, refers to an "escape from reality into fantasy." It was coined relatively recently, at the dawn of the 20th century within the new discipline of psychology, to describe those adults who had difficulty remaining within ordinary consciousness and who tended to withdraw into a more private, hidden world.

By the 1940s and 1950s two psychologists, Leo Kanner and Hans Asperger, almost simultaneously came across children who exhibited a similar "flight from reality," seeming to withdraw from the world of the senses to an inner world hidden from the outside observer. They were not mentally deficient, though they could easily be mistaken for such, living in a vastly different world from the people around them.

Because the term had previously referred to adults, this new condition was termed "early infantile autism." Since the current focus is on the unprecedented increase in an autistic-like condition in children, the shortened form, autism, has come to be more commonly used. Fewer than 50 years ago the original incidence was reported as 1:10,000, a rarity. The frequency of autism is now at 15:10,000, representing an astronomical increase of 15,000%. When polio struck in the 1950's, a series of epidemics were declared when more than 20 children per 100,000 were affected. At this level, paralytic polio was considered a public health disaster that mobilized the resources of the Western world.[1]

What is happening to our children? Along with this dramatic increase in autism, from past medical curiosity to common occurrence, we have also witnessed a plethora of children's behavioral conditions, known popularly by their initials, such as ADD, ADHD, PDD and ODD. A doctor in Virginia reported only a few years ago that almost 90% of her young

---

[1] Before 1955, an outbreak of polio was considered to be of epidemic proportion when 20 or more cases of polio occurred per 100,000 population. The definition of a polio epidemic, again, coincident with the introduction of the Salk vaccine, was changed to 35 cases of polio per 100,000 population, within a one-year period.

(from http://www.worldchiropracticalliance.org/tcj/1989/aug/aug1989g.htm - The Chiropractic Journal)

patients have a form of autism. It's as if the infectious diseases of the 19th and early 20th century, which struck with such ferocity at those under five, have been replaced with these modern "psychological" conditions (see statistics at http://www.healthsentinel.com). The incidence curve of behavioral disorders is strikingly similar to the past infectious disease curves of scarlet fever, diphtheria, whooping cough, etc.

What has been the response of conventional physicians? Official medicine has been able to provide a description of the condition, but has effectively been rendered impotent when it comes to treatment. This is not that far removed from the state of medicine at the start of the modern drug era, when the famous physician, Dr. William Osler, showed a graduating class of doctors a medical textbook of a century earlier, noting that it was long on description and woefully short on any effective treatment, adding that since then nothing had really changed. Dr. Osler would feel right at home today, if a little dismayed at the current state of medical knowledge regarding early infantile autism.

The modern lay definition of autism in children, as formulated by the Autism Society of America, is simply descriptive:

> AUTISM is a severely incapacitating lifelong developmental disability that typically appears during the first three years of life. It occurs in approximately fifteen out of every 10,000 births and is four times more common in boys than girls. It has been found throughout the world in families of all racial, ethnic and social backgrounds. No known factors in the psychological environment of a child have been shown to cause autism.
>
> Autism occurs by itself or in association with other disorders that affect the function of the brain such as viral infections, metabolic disturbances, and epilepsy. It is important to distinguish autism from retardation or mental disorders since diagnostic confusion may result in referral to inappropriate and ineffective treatment techniques. The severe form of the syndrome may include extreme self-injurious, repetitive, highly unusual and aggressive behavior.

The medical definition is perhaps more detailed, but no more helpful in identifying the cause and effective treatment.

From the *Diagnostic and Statistical Manual of Mental Disorders*, Fourth Edition (DSM IV):

Diagnostic Criteria for 299.00 Autistic Disorder

A. A total of six (or more) items from (1), (2), and (3), with at least two from (1), and one each from (2) and (3)

(1) qualitative impairment in social interaction, as manifested by at least two of the following:

a) marked impairments in the use of multiple nonverbal behavior such as eye-to-eye gaze, facial expression, body posture, and gestures to regulate social interaction

b) failure to develop peer relationships appropriate to developmental level

c) a lack of spontaneous seeking to share enjoyment, interests, or achievements with other people, (e.g., by a lack of showing, bringing, or pointing out objects of interest to other people)

d) lack of social or emotional reciprocity. Note: in the description, it gives the following as examples: not actively participating in simple social play or games, preferring solitary activities, or involving others in activities only as tools or "mechanical" aids.

(2) qualitative impairments in communication as manifested by at least one of the following:

a) delay in, or total lack of, the development of spoken language (not accompanied by an attempt to compensate through alternative modes of communication such as gesture or mime)

b) in individuals with adequate speech, marked impairment in the ability to initiate or sustain a conversation with others

c) stereotyped and repetitive use of language of idiosyncratic language

d) lack of varied, spontaneous make-believe play or social imitative play appropriate to developmental level

(3) restricted repetitive and stereotyped patterns of behavior, interests and activities, as manifested by at least two of the following:

a) encompassing preoccupation with one or more stereotyped and restricted patterns of interest that is abnormal either in intensity or focus

b) apparently inflexible adherence to specific, nonfunctional routines or rituals

c) stereotyped and repetitive motor mannerisms (e.g., hand or finger flapping or twisting, or complex whole-body movements)

d) persistent preoccupation with parts of objects

B. Delays or abnormal functioning in at least one of the following areas, with onset prior to age 3 years:

(1) social interaction

(2) language as used in social communication

(3) symbolic or imaginative play

C. The disturbance is not better accounted for by Rett's Disorder or Childhood Disintegrative Disorder

Autism and PDD

From the Autism Society of America (www.autism-society.org)

Diagnosing Autism, PDD, or Asperger's Disorder

The term "PDD" is widely used by professionals to refer to children with autism and related disorders; however, there is a great deal of disagreement and confusion among professionals concerning the PDD label. Diagnosis of PDD, Autism, or any other developmental disability, is based upon the Diagnostic and Statistical Manual of Mental Disorders - Fourth Edition (DSM-IV), published by the American Psychiatric Association, Washington D.C., 1994, the main diagnostic reference of Mental Health professionals in the United States of America.

According to the DSM-IV, the term "PDD" is not a specific diagnosis, but an umbrella term under which the following specific diagnoses are defined:

- Autistic Disorder
- Rett's Disorder
- Childhood Disintegrative Disorder
- Asperger's Disorder
- Pervasive Developmental Disorder Not Otherwise Specified (PDD-NOS)

Diagnostic labels are used to indicate commonalities among individuals. The diagnosis of autism indicates the existence of qualitative impairments in communication, social skills, and range of interests and activities. As no medical tests can be performed to indicate the presence of autism or any other PDD, the diagnosis is based upon the presence or absence of specific behaviors. For example, a child may be diagnosed as having PDD-NOS if he or she has some behaviors that are seen in autism, but does not meet the full criteria for having autism. Most importantly, whether a child is diagnosed with PDD, PDD-NOS, or autism, his or her treatment will be similar.

Reported "Causes" of Autism

Autism in children has been linked to many triggers or causes, from lack of parental love and nurturing, to chemicals in food, to vaccinations and inherited factors. Here is a list of suspected "causes":

- Yeast infections
- Intolerance to specific food substances
- Gluten intolerance ("Leaky Gut Syndrome"/Casein intolerance) causing intestinal permeability and allowing improperly digested peptides to enter the bloodstream and cross the blood-brain barrier
- Phenolsulphertransferase (PST) deficiency
- Brain injury
- Constitutional vulnerability
- Developmental aphasia
- Deficits in the reticular activating system
- Structural cerebellar changes
- Genetic causes
- Viral causes
- Immunological ties
- Vaccines
- Seizures
- Heavy metal toxicity

Conventional medicine still seems to vacillate between a psychological (behavioral) and a biological explanation of early infantile autism. There is no single theory of the cause of autism that is convincing, and it is commonly accepted that there are multiple causes. Some parents of autistic children fit an autistic parent personality profile, but others don't. Siblings of autistic children are invariably non-autistic.

Treatment has been equally disparate, with no standard approach. It mainly focuses on four areas:

- Biochemical e.g., food allergies, drugs, food and vitamin supplements
- Neurosensory e.g., sensorial integration, over-stimulation and patterning, auditory training, facilitated communication, daily life therapy
- Psycho-dynamic e.g., holding therapy, psychotherapy and psychoanalysis
- Behavioral e.g., behavior modification

There is no one drug that has been shown to be consistently successful in treating the *symptoms*, much less getting at the *cause*. In some cases the drugs produce negative results beyond even the usual expected "side-effects" which is a covert way of saying unwanted disease-engendering effects. The list of drugs used or tried is quite impressive, in contrast to the results:

- Desipramine (tricyclic antidepressant)
- Ritalin (methylphenidate) - one of a group of stimulants which include amphetamine, amantidine and fenfluramine
- Dexedrine, an amphetamine used to treat ADD and ADHD in the same way as Ritalin
- Anafranil (cloripramine - a tricyclic antidepressant)
- SRRI "Selective Serotonin Reuptake Inhibitor" drugs, a class of psychoactive drugs that includes Prozac fluoxetine, Zoloft, Luvox (fluxovamine), and Paxil (paroxetine)
- Clomipramine (anti-depressant)
- Clonidine (anti-hypertensive used to settle ADD and ADHD children)
- Dilantin (phenytoin – an anti-convulsive)
- Lithium (for bi-polar disorders)
- Naltrexone (oral version of naloxone – a narcotic antagonist)
- Haldol (haloperidol – a neuroleptic used in psychosis)
- Prednisone (steroid)

- Tegretol (anti-convulsant)
- Nizoral (ketaconazole – anti-fungal)
- Nystatin (anti-fungal)

The Frustration

It's hard to escape the conclusion that medicine, at least the official version, is thrashing around in the dark while facing an epidemic of biblical proportions for children in the Western world. The failure of official or conventional medicine to provide either a convincing theoretical explanation of the cause, or any effective treatment, has left parents and other family members with the burden of seeking help elsewhere. What they face is a Herculean task.

It's not simply a matter of finding enough money to afford "alternative" treatment, much of it not covered by insurance, nor of helping to raise money for research with the hope of an eventual cure. It is trying to work in an environment that fails to understand and address the deeper meaning and causes of the high incidence of autistic behavior.

A Mis-Understanding of Disease

The problem lies in the failure of conventional medicine to understand *true* disease and illness. Autism is a description of a set of behavioral traits, and is not a diagnosis of a disease. A true diagnosis both identifies the cause or origin *and* the remedial medicine or therapeutic modality needed to correct the disease or imbalance. This is what the term diagnosis originally meant in the medical context. It comes from the Greek words "dia" (by, or through) and "gnosis" (knowledge). The lack of a true diagnosis bars the way to an effective treatment approach. The problem, in medical terms, is not the behavior, but what is *producing or causing* the behavior.

The unconventional medical, or natural health field, has perhaps had more success than conventional medicine in the treatment of autism, but here again there is the same failure to understand the nature of disease, leaving the results inconsistent, unfocused and often superficial and not long-lasting. When there *are* individual successes, which any approach *can* claim, they become miracles because we don't understand how they happened, but the same approaches don't seem to work in the vast majority of cases. If the approach is not *easily reproducible through clearly defined principles*, it is of little value. A true system of medicine is not about miracles, but should provide consistent success according to known principles of natural law.

Some children will experience a reduction in symptomology by using Vitamin B_6 in large doses; some to eliminating dairy and/or gluten; others to sound therapy (Auditory Integration Training), Sensory Integration Therapy or Holding Therapy; and still others to dimethyl amino ethanol (found abundantly in fish); or cranio-sacral therapy. There are more than 300 different alternative therapies for the treatment of autism and a large number have, no doubt, been tried by some parents and in some cases found to be successful. Most parents are left to try that which seemed to work for the child of a friend, acquaintance or support group member, but with otherwise very little guidance.

What We Need

What we need are fewer individual "miracles," (being events that occur according to natural law but the basis of which is unknown to us) and more *true science* (conscious knowledge of the use and application of nature's laws). We need an approach to medicine that is able to act *effectively* and *consistently* according to the natural and cosmic laws underpinning disease and health. Only then will we enter a world where autism is no longer a mystery and a subject of fear, but a medical condition whose causes are understood and, thus, are open to effective removal.

What we face, then, in an effort to understand the cause and meaning of "early infantile autism" is the need for a more rational and scientific approach to disease identification. This is the first objective of this book.

It is dedicated to all parents and caregivers who have made the long, difficult and frustrating journey on their own, often with little help or direction from conventional medical authorities, and without much more from the so-called alternative health field.

The problem lies not in the intentions, nor in the dedication of individuals, but as so often in the history of science, from a limitation in what Thomas Kuhn, a physicist turned historian, called the prevailing paradigm or model that governs and limits thinking in any given era. What we see and hear is limited by this paradigm. Most, if not all, scientific discovery comes from outside the prevailing paradigm by those who have not been steeped in its view of the world and who can see that the Emperor has no clothes.

Our current paradigm of health, disease, illness and therapeutics is seriously flawed despite the technological advances in emergency medicine; the current plague of children's behavioral conditions is making this painfully obvious.

Format of This Book

The first part of this book sets out a radically different understanding of disease and illness within which autism can be understood, along with virtually any disturbance of health. It also provides an effective and consistent means of removal of the disease(s) underlying autism in children.

At the same time, it is not enough to identify disease correctly; we also need, as practitioners and parents, to understand the meaning of autism. Without meaning, we will remain in the negative phase of health-care, namely, getting rid of unwanted symptoms. However, this does not address the deeper wounds of society, those within the families and communities touched by this modern phenomenon. In more traditional societies, it was not sufficient to remove disease and heal the individual; disease was recognized as involving forces that touched on the spiritual realms of man, both individually and collectively. The typical health issues of a generation or era say much about the deeper issues we need to come to terms with as human beings. This theme is much more difficult to discern at this stage, but some thoughts will be given for reflection in the second part of this book.

The third part of the book gives actual case histories, spread through the book, to illustrate the principles of this new understanding of disease – new in the sense of not being generally known and only recently more fully and consciously developed. However, its principles and origins go back to antiquity and are grounded in natural law. This is not to say that any given approach to treatment has not provided successes, or sometimes even dramatic reversals. Indeed, they have. However, they are inconsistent, and there is much misunderstanding as to *why* what works in one case does *not* work in so many other cases of autism.

The model presented in this book, termed Heilkunst, provides such an insight, at least to a greater degree than hitherto known. Heilkunst, in its identification of disease, is disclosive rather than simply discursive (descriptive). It provides knowledge of disease that is powerful in its ability to go inside "autism" and provide an effective treatment based on causes, rather than simply describing what is happening and treating the symptoms.

Autism Facts from the Autism Society of America

1 in 250 births
1 to 1.5 million Americans
Fastest-growing developmental disability
10 - 17 % annual growth

Growth comparison during the 1990s:

U.S. population increase: 13%
Disabilities increase: 16%
Autism increase: 172%

$90 billion annual cost
90% of costs are in adult services

Sebastien's Story

Sebastien had officially been diagnosed with autism when he was three years old, but his parents felt that he could have been diagnosed much earlier, at the age of 18 months. He was nine when he started treatment with us.

Several days after his very first remedies to remove a dental trauma, plus to help his system process emotional stresses, Sebastien had a strong healing reaction that worsened his hyperactive state and sleep difficulties, but he then fell into a "beautiful sleep pattern." His obsessions moderated somewhat as well, and he had a greater desire to be with his siblings, which was new.

It was interesting that his teeth also became brownish in color, which pointed to his previous trauma (going backwards chronologically), namely his many rounds of antibiotics. After treating next for the antibiotics, Sebastien's attention improved, his sleep continued to be great and his hyperactivity lessened. His teeth turned black and he started obsessing about toilets.

We increased the strength of his emotional remedies and his constitutional drops, and then treated for various drugs that he had been prescribed. His physical state improved dramatically in terms of appetite (even eating beef, which he had never done before) to the extent that he actually put on muscle mass. His father reported that where he had always shivered in water, even in the summer, he now could go in without any problem. His teeth had turned yellow.

Emotionally, his giggling worsened, but overall he was more stable, more aware or the emotional needs of others, and could recall and communicate things for the first time. His father reported that he had "tidbits of beautiful language" and an emerging sense of humor, though his attention span was still short.

After the next treatment, his teeth turned white for a period, then yellow again, and there were further cognitive advances, as well as greater language skills, including jokes. Then, following another treatment to remove antibiotics and sulpha drugs, his obsessions decreased even further, his social skills increased and he showed greater cognitive abilities and language skills.

Next was the removal of the shock of a DPTP/Hi(b) vaccination, which resulted in a strong healing reaction (an emotional breakdown and crying). He suddenly developed an obsession with cutting shirts and became afraid of toilets. These improved over the month though, along with his language and social skills.

Just prior to the next treatment he drew a picture of a boy in a crib with a huge syringe in his arm, and interestingly, the next remedies to be prescribed were for the shock of his MMR vaccination. During the month Sebastien's obsessive-compulsive behavior increased, he began toe-walking for the first time and wanted three to four baths each day. He also became obsessed with toilet flushing and breaking glasses. According to his parents, he developed classic autistic symptoms that he had not had before.

The following month things improved somewhat overall and he stopped toe-walking. By the second month following the MMR treatment, Sebastien was doing very well, was much calmer with better eye contact, greater social skills and improved communication.

Parent's Comments

Sebastien is a ten-year old boy with moderate to severe autistic symptoms. At ten, his speech is delayed and fragmented. His behavior is obsessive-compulsive at times, he either lacks energy or he is hyperactive, and he sleeps poorly, waking several times at night. Despite everything, Sebastien has shown a great deal of improvement since we started Heilkunst.

He was diagnosed at three because of a lack of language, poor social interaction and repetitive play. He has received Applied Behavioral Analysis since then. While ABA has played a significant role in his learning, it became evident to us fairly early in the game that he was missing something. We call this the veil of autism. Strangely enough, it wasn't a question of intelligence. We found out that he was very intelligent when he was highly motivated to do something. He was good at some things, and very poor at others. Worse yet, the good/poor things changed from one week to the next. His brain was like Swiss cheese.

When he turned five, we started assuming that his autism was associated with a medical condition. We had read about the effect of dietary intervention, vitamin supplementation, gut yeast infection, food allergies and/or intolerances and mercury poisoning. Sebastien tested positive for all these and we worked toward improving his health. After four years of naturopathic intervention his health had improved considerably but it was evident that there was a deeper factor involved in Sebastien's autism. Sebastien continued to make steady progress under ABA, but there was nothing spectacular.

We became interested in the Heilkunst method progressively. We had used off the shelf homeopathic remedies for years to deal with acute conditions such as headaches, bee stings, indigestion and the broad array of hurts a family of five comes up with. Looking deeper, we became fascinated with the concept of reverse detoxification and miasms. Both made a great deal of sense. On the one hand, we had seen Sebastien's health decline progressively since his birth. He had reacted poorly to his inoculations. On the other hand, we had read about chronic miasms as the bio-energetic equivalent of the genetic codes. With accumulated chronic miasms, the chance of autism was greater where they were weak or non-existent. As far as Sebastien was concerned both sets of grandparents showed conditions that could contribute to autism.

We started Heilkunst's reverse detoxification of shocks and traumas, particularly vaccinations, with an open mind and minimal expectations. After all, six years of battling the dragons of autism tends to turn anyone, even the most optimistic among us, into skeptics. However, we quickly saw a strong correlation between those things we were detoxing for and healing reactions in the form of a temporary return of the symptoms we had seen in the past. Treatment for antibiotics in the past, for example, caused rashes and diarrhea, which we had seen many times over. Along with those physical symptoms, we saw Sebastien cycle in and out of the symptoms of autism. When we detoxed him for his DPT shots he became withdrawn and was covered with rashes.

A week before Sebastien was to start the removal of the shock from his twelve-month MMR shots he drew the picture which covers this book. It was a spontaneous drawing that stunned everyone. Sebastien was reliving his twelve-month shots. For the skeptics, no one outside of me knew for what Sebastien was being treated. It is important to add that Sebastien had reacted very poorly to his twelve-month shots. He had high bouts of fever, sat on the couch and stared at nothing for hours. We were really scared then. Therefore, it made sense that we should have had expected a strong reaction to the MMR shots. I concede that I cannot prove that Sebastien was made autistic by inoculations. However, I'm positive that they contributed to the deterioration of his health.

Soon after the completion of the reverse detox protocol we had Sebastien's health tested. To our complete amazement he came up healthier than anybody else in the family. We took this as evidence that the reverse detox has had a clear positive impact on his health. We also noted that his language and attention had improved significantly. Others also remarked on these changes.

As I write this note, Sebastien has gone through two treatments for the chronic miasms, each time a little deeper, and each time we have seen him temporarily withdraw behind the veil of autism and then come back yet stronger, more in tune with our world and with a better control of his emotions and behaviors. One issue that was of particular concern was his fear. Among many things he was afraid of monsters and dogs. The fear of monsters kept him awake at night. The sight of a dog put him into a panic.

There wasn't much we could do about monsters, except treat this as part of a miasm. However, his fear of dogs gave us a good marker for success. We treated his fear with different potencies of *Stramonium*. Eventually we borrowed a dog from friends and brought it home. To our surprise we found Sebastien lying on the couch, using the dog as a pillow. We saw this as a tremendous step forward and we bought a dog, which turned out to be a wonderful companion for Sebastien. He now goes to bed with the door to his bedroom shut. He loves taking the dog for a walk.

Sebastien might need another two or three years of Heilkunst to fully recover, if it is possible at all. However, of all the treatment programs we have used, Heilkunst has proven to be the most beneficial.

2| Heilkunst: A Comprehensive Model of Health and Disease

The contention of this book is that autism is not a disease in its own right, but a set of symptoms that have been lumped together and given a name that is simply descriptive (and not necessarily accurate) rather than disclosive of its cause and cure. This is the situation with so much of modern, conventional medicine, but equally so with respect to the natural health field.

The autistic condition is only the result of one or more diseases in a person that must, in each individual case, be identified and sequentially removed. Identifying the diseases behind a given case requires a different nosological (disease-classification) understanding from that which prevails in conventional or unconventional medicine.

A Primer on Disease and Health

Conventional Medical Treatment

When it comes to understanding *why* we get sick, it seems we are pretty much in the dark and have made little progress since the time of Hippocrates. Instead of some unnamed evil spirit, now we are told we are suffering from some named or unnamed "virus," and that there is not much that can be done. Or we are given a "diagnosis" in the form of some arbitrary and vague disease name and are prescribed one or more drugs to control the symptoms. Research money continues to fund the search for ever-elusive cures, but when it comes to treatment, medicine is purely a game of suppression of symptoms.

Rather than a health-care system, we have more of a "disease-management" system. Blood pressure pills control the blood pressure (though not always), and stomach pills control the acid reflux (though not always), and painkillers control the migraines (though not always), and the patient has to keep taking the pills or the problem returns, and meanwhile his or her overall level of health declines.

Although you might be grateful for some temporary relief, you will likely suffer from chronic problems due to the unwanted disease-engendering power of chemical drugs (so-called "side-effects"), which may or may not be worse than the original symptoms.

One case we had in our clinic illustrates this very well. A woman in her sixties was suffering from high blood pressure and a host of other symptoms like fatigue, depression, stomach pains and constipation. Originally she had been prescribed anti-hypertensives for a sudden high blood pressure problem. This medication produced stomach discomfort, which was addressed with another drug, which in turn produced new symptoms to be addressed by yet another drug. In fewer than six years the patient had accumulated some 14 different drug prescriptions – one to treat the original problem, the others to treat the iatrogenic (doctor-caused) diseases!

Rather than simply treating the symptoms caused by the drugs, we sought to discover the original cause of the high blood pressure, which had led to the unfortunate state of our patient. On questioning we learned that she had suffered the increase in blood pressure immediately following her husband's sudden death. We addressed the shock of his death and within two weeks her blood pressure had returned to normal, which it had never done while she was on medication. She was then able to stop taking all of her drugs and regain her previous state of health.

Most patients eventually realize that chemical drugs only suppress their symptoms. They may appreciate the relief initially, but are fully aware that the original cause of their symptoms remains. It seems that conventional medicine is good at getting rid of the evidence, but more in the manner of sweeping it under the carpet. It also comes with a massive price tag, not only in terms of the direct cost in dollars, but indirectly in terms of the impact of drug treatment on health. Iatrogenic disease (disease caused by doctors themselves, including their prescriptions) is the leading cause of death in North America today.

Stop the Allopathic Merry-Go-Round, I Want to Get Off!

Once you have stepped off the merry-go-round of conventional medicine, you are faced with a bewildering array of alternative therapies and products, each promising to make you well and each with testimonials of cured cases. How can they all promise to fix your ailment, and why doesn't the one that worked for your friend's child work for yours? How do you know which one to choose?

We had often wondered this ourselves. Our search for answers led us to Heilkunst, a logical, rational, truly scientific *system of medicine*. It has allowed us to answer these questions about disease and illness for our patients and for ourselves.

What is Heilkunst?

Heilkunst is a little known, yet powerful system of remediation based on natural law and scientific principles. The German term comes from two words – *heil*, which has the dual meaning of "cure and healing," and *kunst*, which means "the art." Thus, at a very simple level the word Heilkunst has the basic meaning of "the medical art," but in its deepest sense means the rational approach to making people whole human beings at *all* levels – body, mind, soul and spirit.

The term *heil* comes from the same root as the Anglo-Saxon word "hale," as in "hale and hearty." Heilkunst seeks to remove disease using natural law and to restore balance, so that our innate life force can be used for the higher, spiritual purposes of our existence on earth. In essence, each life has meaning, and each life is a journey back to self, enriched and further evolved from the struggle of our human condition. Our diseases and our illnesses are the context for this journey and give it meaning.

Disease Versus Imbalance

The basis of all understanding is precise terminology. We tend to toss words around like confetti and think one is just a synonym for another, particularly words like sick, ill, disease and imbalance.

When you're not feeling well or your child is sick, words aren't that important – you just want to feel better or for your child to stop suffering. But words are critical, even vital, to successful treatment. To be sick and to be ill are two very different things. All sick people are ill, but not all ill people are sick. Disease and illness are different, as we explain below.

Dual Nature of the Life Force

We have a living principle within us, a dynamic power that animates us, digests our lunch, keeps us healthy, allows us to think and allows us to grow, learn, change and create. This living force or power, which is called the *Dynamis*, has two aspects, almost like Siamese twins. All cultures and traditions have a term for this living, dynamic power – chi, prana, etc. What is not often realized or emphasized is the dual nature of this life force and the importance that this plays in understanding and effectively treating illness and disease.

One side of the Dynamis simply tries to maintain a state of health. That's its job, and it has a one-track mind. When you lose your health, it goes to work to restore balance. We call this the *sustentive power* of the Dynamis, as it sustains us in health.

The other side of the Dynamis allows our cells to divide, allows us to generate something new – an idea, a child, a work of art. We call this the *generative power* for obvious reasons.

Why is this distinction important? For one thing, it allows us to understand the vital distinction between simply being ill and being sick. Being ill means that you are out of balance.

When the sustentive power is off balance you feel ill, and your sense of well-being is diminished. Your normal functions and processes are not working properly because you have an absolute excess or lack of something, or simply too much of something in one part of the body and not enough in another.

Imbalance

Let's assume that you don't get enough Vitamin C in your diet. You start to feel a little tired, you feel the symptoms of a viral infection coming on or your eyes become sore and bloodshot. If you simply take some Vitamin C the sustentive power is then able to restore balance. The problem, the lack of Vitamin C, is solved. There is no *disease*, just an imbalance in your normal homeostasis ("balance") that needs to be addressed. To supply the missing Vitamin C is a simple, yet profound solution, based on the natural law of opposites (*contraria contrariis*) known from earliest times. It's a natural law because unlike human law, it doesn't change.

Disease

Disease is a very different matter from illness. Disease exists when some external agent or event affects (impinges upon in some way) our generative power. This can be due to a toxin, a drug or vaccination, an emotional or physical shock or an infectious disease agent. Instead of simply creating an imbalance in the sustentive power, these events damage the *generative* power and create a limit on the restoration of health, which *cannot* be addressed by altering the *quantity* of something according to the law of opposites, like taking more vitamin C.

This damage or impingement is akin to what occurs in pregnancy. No amount of exercise, healthy food, supplements or rest is going to remove the pregnancy, or the state of impregnation. We recognize that the process of impregnation can occur at other than the physical level ("pregnant with ideas"). This impregnation of the generative power occurs classically in the case of the truly infectious diseases, like measles, but can occur in other cases as well, like from shocks involving drugs, vaccinations, emotional traumas, etc. We need to reverse the process, like reverse time-lapse photography. How can this be done?

The Natural Law of Similars

We saw that the sustentive power is able to restore balance in the case of imbalance when we use the natural law of opposites. But if there is damage to the generative side of the Dynamis, this will not work. Use of therapies that support the sustentive power can make us feel better, can strengthen our energy and constitution, but it can't remove the damage to our generative power caused by disease. Cure of disease requires the application of a remedy, in this case a medicine that is applied according to the other natural law of treatment – the law of *similars*.

The law of similars involves, seemingly paradoxically, the use of a medicine that, if used on a healthy person, would produce a similar disease or disease symptoms in that person. For example, if your eyes get irritated from cutting onions, you can cure it by taking a very minute dose of specially prepared onion (*Allium cepa*).

Let's say you touch some poison ivy and get a rash with intense itching. You can simply take a small, highly diluted and energized dose of poison ivy (*Rhus tox*) to cure it. This can even act preventively. Pioneers, who were busy clearing the land and always at risk of poison ivy, learned to drink a tea in the spring made from young poison ivy leaves. The tea protected them from reacting to poison ivy all season. This is an example of the law of similars.

But the law of similars goes beyond this. If someone complains of vomiting and diarrhea, has a strong need for fresh air but is freezing despite being piled under the covers, and has a lot of fear or anxiety, this presents a picture of arsenic poisoning. The person swears, reasonably enough, that they have not ingested arsenic, but it certainly looks as if they had. We would say the person is suffering from an "arsenic-like" disease. The law of similars justifies our giving the person an energized, diluted dose of arsenic (*Arsenicum album*), which will cure the symptoms.

We had a dramatic case of a woman who called us at 3:00 a.m. from Mexico City with a sudden case of dysentery. She had continual diarrhea and vomiting, was restless and very anxious. The symptoms and the situation matched that of an "arsenic-like" disease.

Luckily she had an emergency homeopathic remedy kit with her. We told her to dissolve a few pellets of *Arsenicum* in water and to sip it every few minutes until her symptoms subsided. She told us on her return that she felt better within minutes, and within an hour her symptoms had gone and she was able to sleep.

By morning she was almost fully recovered, needing only to drink some extra fluids and restore lost electrolytes. The extra fluids and electrolyte replacement placed her back in the realm of the law of opposites, since once the disease had been removed using the law of similars we needed to help her sustentive power restore balance or homeostasis.

Two Sides of Disease

Next we look at another important distinction, the one between the disease itself, and the body's efforts to get *rid* of disease. This means that disease has two sides or aspects: the initial action of the *disease* agent that dynamically affects the generative power, causing the impingement, and then the *counteraction* by the sustentive power of the Dynamis as it seeks to restore balance.

Let's take a simple case of an infectious disease, like chickenpox. Your child goes to a friend's house and a few days later the mother calls to tell you that her child has broken out with the characteristic eruptions of chickenpox. We all know that the neighbor's child was infectious for a week to ten days prior to the rash appearing, so now you can expect that your child will come down with visible symptoms of chickenpox in a week or so.

Your child *already* has the disease, which means in turn that the generative power is already infected by the chickenpox microbe. Yet, your child doesn't have any symptoms at this point; these come later. *Why*?

Remember the sustentive power, the one whose job it is to keep you in health? It starts to make preparations to repel the invader. First it has to marshal its resources, get its lines of communication clear and prepare the different parts of the immune system to do battle. Then it goes into action. It's this reaction of the sustentive power to the disease itself that produces the characteristic fever, followed by the itching and rash, as well as a general feeling of lassitude, that we suffer and commonly *call* the disease. It's part of the whole disease process, but *not* of the disease.

Chronic Disease and Healing Reactions

Why is this important to know, you might ask? It becomes important when we look at the process of cure and healing (remediation) in the case of chronic disease.

Up until now we have used examples of simple disease cases, but what if it's not so simple, which is most often the case these days? Chickenpox will go away on its own eventually, even if you don't do anything. It is an example of what we call self-limiting diseases.

Diseases that don't go away on their own, however, are called chronic diseases. Unless they are removed, these types of diseases continue inexorably, until you die. They require careful identification so they can be destroyed. And when the right remedy is given on the basis of the law of similars, the disease *is* destroyed, not simply suppressed. This is a very gentle action.

The sustentive power of the Dynamis is then roused to *react to* the curative action of the medicine. This counter action, called the *healing reaction*, can involve a number of general symptoms, such as changes in temperature, mood, disturbances of sleep, and various discharge reactions at the physical level (nausea, mucous discharge, perspiration, etc.). This healing reaction is not always pleasant, but is followed by a general feeling of increased well-being and soundness as well as an improvement in the disease symptoms about which the patient was initially complaining.

Healing Reaction vs. Counteraction

A critical part of the training of a physician should be in the process of distinguishing the important healing reaction phase of a remedial process from the counter-action of a disease process. They can appear very similar to the untrained eye. Conventional doctors are trained to see *all* symptoms as part of a disease process and, therefore, treat disease and remedial symptoms the same – as something to be countered and suppressed.

The healing reaction can be likened to a home renovation. In the process of restoring the "health" of an old house, the state of the house appears to be worse – old cabinets ripped out, floors torn up, windows removed, etc. The homeowners aren't concerned because they understand what a renovation involves and "see," in the seeming mess, the underlying truth that their home will be greatly improved at the end despite appearances to the contrary.

Let's imagine, however, that you have a visitor who comes from a planet where people don't have a concept of renovation because their homes never deteriorate, they are perpetually perfect.

He comes to earth to visit you and, when he gets to your home, calls the police because he sees people tearing apart your roof and otherwise appearing to vandalize your home. He assumes the renovators are vandalizing your house because he has no frame of reference to understand anything else. The police come while you are at work, arrest the workers and the renovation (healing) comes to a halt. This is the situation you are in when you see a doctor or anyone else in the health field who doesn't understand the concept of a healing reaction.

Almost all symptoms of discomfort are seen as a disease process. These, in his eyes, must be *opposed*, so that most conventional measures involve *antipathic* medicines (which are based on the natural law of opposites), that is, measures that *suppress* the symptoms of the healing reaction (anti-inflammatories, anti-biotics, anti-depressants, anti-histamines, etc.). Since the symptoms of healing are seen as negative, suppression becomes, in this context, positive.

However, suppression of the body's efforts at healing only weakens the overall state of health of the patient. It may provide relief from the discomfort of the healing reaction, but this relief comes at a price. Let's look at the case of inflammation.

The Role of Inflammation in Healing

The body's way of healing is to generate an inflammatory process, which marshals the resources of the immune and repair systems and directs them to a particular area of weakness or damage. The body also produces its own bacteria to clean up the dead and dying tissue, much as the oil industry now uses beneficial bacteria to clean up an oil spill. This inflammatory process produces some pain and discomfort, but then results in a greater level of health and functioning, similar to the home renovation.

However, antibiotics and anti-inflammatories, even cold applications on a sprain or a strain, are designed to *shut down* this process. Blocking a natural repair process and the necessary clean-up of toxins can only *weaken*, not strengthen.

This is graphically illustrated by the child we were treating for a weak immune system (constant colds), with chronic earaches and allergy symptoms. On a regular visit to the pediatrician during the process of treatment, he noticed some redness in his ears.

The child had not complained of pain or discomfort at all, yet this inflammatory process, actually part of the healing reaction to some natural remedies the child was taking, was assumed by the pediatrician to be an infection. No actual test for bacterial infection was done, which is also all too common, and he prescribed antibiotics. The mother still accepted (at that point) that inflammation = infection, and infection meant that antibiotics had to be used.

After the child was on antibiotics for several days the mother noticed that his appetite was not the same and that he was showing some signs of unusual crankiness. Overall, he did not seem as healthy as he had been previously. She returned to the doctor in a week and the redness was still there. A second round of antibiotics was prescribed although the mother had reported the negative effects, which concerned her.

During the second course of antibiotics the mother noticed her son becoming even more lethargic and irritable and that he had trouble walking, which was very unusual. She returned to the pediatrician after a week and the redness was still present in the ear. Despite the mother's concern the doctor prescribed a third round of antibiotics.

That straw broke the camel's back – she lost faith in the conventional treatment and brought the child to our clinic. We explained that the redness was a healing reaction. We treated for the shock of the antibiotics on the child's system and within a few days he had recovered to his previous state of health. The redness eventually disappeared on its own after the healing process had been completed. Since then the child has been in good health.

Internal and External Microbes

Despite technological advances conventional medicine is still based on the simplistic 19th century premise of Louis Pasteur that the body is aseptic (has no microbes) and that any microbe found in the body has to have come from *outside* - an unwanted invader. The search for the cause of disease is still very much the search for a bacteria or virus of some sort. It's true that certain diseases *are* caused by infectious external microbes, such as malaria, cholera, yellow fever or typhoid, but there are many diseases, mainly the chronic, degenerative diseases, that have *no* microbial cause.

However, these chronic disease states alter the level of health to such a degree that the body starts to change its makeup. Initially, the body will produce, as we saw, bacteria to *help* in the repair process. If this is not successful the body is weakened and starts to die prematurely. This process produces internal viruses and fungi, most commonly seen in the cases of systemic candidiasis.

Polymorphic Nature of Microbes

While conventional medicine latched on to Pasteur's rather simple notion that each microbial form is unique, other researchers, who took the trouble to observe microbes for extended periods of time, argued with convincing evidence that a microbe could change form under altered conditions of health. This is termed the polymorphic view, from the Greek term "many forms."

What they discovered was that the body itself would produce many different microbial forms when it was stressed. The more stressed it was, the more the body would produce viral and fungal forms as opposed to bacterial forms. These microbes were not the *cause* of any disease, but rather the *result.*

Supporters of the polymorphic view placed the emphasis of treatment on the underlying state of health of the body, stressing nutrition, hygiene and lifestyle. Further research also showed that bacteria were produced as part of the body's healing reaction; they are the necessary scavengers of the dead tissue that healthy tissue replaces. The use of antibiotics (literally "anti-life" agents) served only to shut down the inflammation and to kill off these beneficial bacteria.

The debate raged in the last part of the 19th and early 20th century between the Pasteurian view and that of his colleague, Antoine Bechamp, as to the origin of disease. Pasteur's view was too rigid. Bechamp's view made allowance for infectious diseases, but also recognized that not all bacterial or viral evidence could be interpreted as the cause of disease.

However, the advent of the patented drug age in the 1940's virtually eliminated any emphasis in conventional medicine on nutrition and lifestyle, and all treatment focused on finding a drug to kill the presumed bacteria or virus. This is also the period in which medical schools and medicine came more and more under the influence of the pharmaceutical conglomerates, which had a vested interest in research for patentable drugs.

Essentially, conventional medicine now assumes that *any* inflammation is an attempt to fight off a microbial invasion and that any microbe found in the body came from outside and is a disease agent. But in order to be objective, conventional medicine must prove three things (called Koch's postulates) before it can term a microbe a cause of disease rather than just a result of a stressed organism:

- it must be able to isolate the microbe;
- culture it outside the body;
- and then inject it into a healthy subject (animal) and cause the same disease in every case.

The problem is that these conditions are seldom fulfilled, as in the case of the so-called Human Immuno-deficiency Virus (HIV), the supposed cause of AIDS (Acquired Immuno-deficiency Syndrome), or the more recent SARS (Sudden Acute Respiratory Syndrome) outbreak. The virus supposedly responsible is *not* found in all people suffering from these conditions and is found in only small quantities where it *has* been isolated. In scientific terms, we *cannot* say that the virus is the cause of the condition. To find two things together is not proof of cause and effect.

For example, if you are found to be present at a number of bank robberies, we cannot, without further proof, say that you are responsible for the robberies. Yet, so strong is the allopathic mind-set that the virus found *must* be the cause that the strict requirements of Koch's postulates are often ignored or loosely applied. The virus, which is really present because the body is under stress, often from pollution, processed food and chemical drugs, is then claimed as the cause.

Since viruses are very difficult to treat because they change rapidly, strong (and costly) drugs are developed to try to control (suppress) the symptoms. These drugs further weaken thc immune system, thus causing a negative spiral of ill-health.

Matt's story

Matt's mother came to us first in 1999 in an interesting way. In desperation she had written a letter to a magazine about her son's condition. He had never been well since the day he was born. His mother felt that five years of allopathic treatment (his entire life) had only amounted to putting band-aids on the symptoms.

A client of ours actually wrote her a letter, saying that the only treatment she knew of that might have any positive results was Heilkunst, and she shared her own story of her son's treatment success, and referred her to one of our online cases at www.heilkunst.com/cases.html.

Matt, who had many attempts at diagnosis, including Asperger's Syndrome, was suffering on many levels. During his gestation there was phenomenal stress on his mother. All of her grandparents died, and there was great financial stress. During his first few months of life, between the vaccinations at two and four months, he was challenged with colic, severe constipation and vomiting.

When he came to us he had daily headaches, stomachaches and nausea; environmental allergies; a chronic cough; recurrent ear and throat infections; chronic conjunctivitis; eczema; and chronic leg pain that began following a DPTP vaccination at age four where he was unable to roll over, move, or stand to urinate and that caused him to scream from the subsequent discomfort.

He later had a tonsillectomy where he almost suffocated, which caused his doctors to discuss the possibility of performing a tracheotomy. This devolved into pneumonia a few months later, followed by a diagnosis of asthma and a prescription for steroid inhalers – at this point, his mom asked about alternative medicine. She said the doctor was enraged at her suggestion.

With gross and fine motor delays, he was supported with physiotherapy, occupational therapy and a learning resource teacher. He was becoming withdrawn in school, cried a lot and was generally hypersensitive, and could not socialize well or run and climb with other children. He told his mother he wasn't sad *all* the time, just *most* of the time. Because he had a huge heart, it set him up for bullying from the other children. His diet? Not extensive – chicken nuggets and fries, macaroni and cheese (though he would gag if they were spirals), and canned tomato soup and crackers that his mom would use to sneak in pureed veggies.

Within two months of starting treatment his conjunctivitis was, according to his mother, "completely gone, better than it has ever been in his life." His headaches were not as bad, the leg aches were down to one day a week, his stomach had hurt only a few times, and he only had asked for the bucket (to vomit) once.

His father and grandmother noticed he was standing taller, was more lighthearted, and for the first time in his life he was standing up for himself, not giving in to others.

In his third month of treatment his mother reported that, "He is so great, I am not sure if he has ever been this great in his life. He said he feels great, nothing hurts, and he has been doing absolutely fantastic. He is still very emotional, and can get stuck on emotional upsets. And usually this is the worst time of the year for his allergies, and it is amazing, this is the best he has ever been."

It is common for people to begin to express their need for the next remedy on their traumatic timeline, especially if it is delayed beyond the time it might normally be given. And this happened with Matt. The week before he had his next appointment he had begun to backslide, and he had been coughing every morning and had eye crusts. The next remedy on his timeline was for the time in his childhood where he had pneumonia, later resulting in asthma, and three months of antibiotics.

The child psychologist had meanwhile discharged him, saying Matt had found resolve with his issues, and that his problems were developmental. He still had a short attention span, would switch tasks constantly, and was stressed in gym with the noise and having to catch balls, among other activities.

At home the suggestion of doing anything, like picking up his clothing or toys, found him overwhelmed to the point of tears. He never had tantrums, and he was so worried about breaking a rule because it would devastate him if his mother said she was disappointed in him.

By his fourth consultation he had been doing very well with his teacher and progressing academically, doing better with math and reading. He loved working one-on-one with the teacher and was headed for academic testing the following day to assess where he needed to be.

Matt showed less sensitivity now to noise and distractions. He had few bouts of sobbing, and was happier than ever. However, he was not good around other children, was too nervous and easily overwhelmed with groups of children, doing better with a 1:1 or 1:2 ratio. He was starting to feel lonely without too many friends to be with.

Over time he just seemed to gain steady ground in terms of his learning, he liked books and wanted to read everything he could. Penmanship was not his strong suit, but his mom did catch him practicing on his own at times. His mother said at one point that he was bursting with joy, that he was coming out on the other side of disease, and that he would run up to her and hug her, saying he loved her.

About 16 months after beginning treatment (this family did not have appointments monthly, but when it seemed to feel like the right time) his mother commented that there had been so many changes over the last year. She said Matt had so much more confidence, that he was riding a two-wheeler without training wheels and was very proud of himself, and that he was doing very well with reading. His printing was still a challenge, but they were increasing expectations and asking him to print one sentence a day.

We had worked previously to eliminate dairy products from his diet, and then once, during this time, he had three glasses of milk in one day. He woke with crusty and puffy eyes, a headache and a cough, and it took three days for that reaction to clear. He had had so much mucous in his system in the past that his mother said they'd run when he sneezed, and that it could even hit his shoelaces.

At the eighteen-month point his mother said he was 180 degrees from where they started. He was doing well, feeling well, had very few headaches, some leg aches, no crusty eyes, some teary days but that was easily helped with an acute emotional remedy. Interestingly, when he had the remedies for his birth and circumcision he complained of pain in his stomach and penis.

They had found a new school for him and while his mom had been feeling apprehensive, he ran into the classroom and chose his desk. He would come home and talk all about his day at school. The occupational therapist recommended a laptop computer to get past his printing problems.

When he was treated with the sycotic miasm, one of those most sensitive to vaccination shock, his mother reported that they had to gently pick his eyelids apart in the mornings. His mother said she had forgotten how horrible his mucous used to be. It literally poured from his eyes and his mucous sneezes would again reach his shoelaces, and he'd come home from school with long streaks dried onto his coat and pants. He complained about pain on urination and said that his penis was itchy (which is interesting since this miasm originated with gonorrhea). He was upset about a relatively small incident one day and was crying about it. When his mother asked why it bothered him so, he replied that he had to cry to let it out or else he would want to hurt himself.

Matt was still having some problems with insomnia and nightmares, and talked and dreamed of death many nights, but his reading improved dramatically, and he earned 100% on a social science paper. He was elated to receive 26/30 on a math test, which was 20 more points than normal for him.

He became quite emotional as he approached the inherited miasm for cancer. He cried each morning when it was time to go to school, and he was very hard on himself. He drew a happy face on his pillow and sheets, and then denied doing it, and "snapped" when his mother told him not to do things like that. He wanted to hit his head into the wall, to put his fist through glass. He cried for hours, and his mother said he was very dramatic. He had been yelling, “Punish me!” all the time, and was very hard on himself when reprimanded.

His long-past leg pain had returned, and was there each night, and his headache and stomachache had returned as well. He was “dying of loneliness,” his mother said, so much an outsider always looking in, wanting so much to be a part of things.

We interrupted his miasmic treatment for major dental work, requiring general anesthesia. Matt “did amazing,” according to his mother. He was afraid, but also proud that he talked about his fear, because in the past he would not have voiced his emotions. He saved his teeth for Show and Tell at school, and recovered very quickly with the help of the remedies.

Following his remedy for the inherited miasm that comes from syphilis he completely stopped wanting to hurt himself, and the morbid dreams and talk disappeared. His behavior improved, he seemed happier, he liked school more and more. He was doing really well in sciences and liked math too, especially the multiplication chart, where he received a 26/26. His confidence soared. His mother said his behavior was outstanding, that he was well-mannered and polite.

With the more potent remedy for the sycotic miasm Matt began holding onto his penis “like it was a reflex” and was humping his teddy bear. He was more sexual than he had been ever before. A remedy to help with the chthonic realm, along with the miasmic remedies for sycosis, cancer and syphilis, eliminated that.

Matt was treated through three rounds of the inherited miasms, seemingly on an upward spiral to health all the while. A year and a half passed before I heard from his mother again, around the time of this writing. Her report:

“Marvelous! Matt is at the top of his game, I have never seen my son so happy. He’s healthy, thriving, he has grown three inches and two or three shoe sizes since August 2004.

He repeats over and over how he is having a great day, he is really happy. He is in a good school, he works very hard there and has a computer to help with his work. He may have the odd headache, but he is marvelous, has absolutely no issues.

He needs less sleep, he jumps from the bed in the mornings and this is the first year I haven't had to dress him in the mornings because he was so tired. He is happy and alive. He wants to help with dinner, help around the house.

He is reading very well, and I realize he will never be a novel kid, preferring to read a camcorder manual or something like that, which he will take to bed. He's never liked TV or superheroes or cartoons, but recently we were looking for books on computer programming, which he is into now. He is even good with relationships now, and they are just flowing.

Physically he is great – he has the odd headache, but no belly aches or leg aches. He is willingly trying bites of different foods. He is still very childlike in some ways, and in others shows a remarkable sense of maturity. I see a light in his eyes that I have never seen before!"

Parent's Story

"We feared our son was having a nervous breakdown. He was seven years old.

Matt was worried and sad most of the time. Socially he was isolated. Academically he couldn't keep up. The many doctors and specialists that had assessed him had come up with many labels: A.D.D., central auditory processing deficits, fine motor delays, gross motor delays, Asperger's and hypotonia.

Surprisingly, these things were not Matt's biggest problems. Physically his little body was screaming for help. Ear, eye throat, and upper respiratory infections were a constant and Matt was perpetually on antibiotics. He suffered with constipation from birth, resulting in painful fissures. Most bothersome was the headache, bellyache and leg pain. For lack of better treatment he took Tylenol on a daily basis.

His constant cough would rack his pale, thin body, often making sleep impossible. Cough medicine didn't work, and we often had to resort to the emergency room for the steroid mask. When puffers were added three times a day, "...most likely for the rest of his life," we knew there had to be another way.

It would be two more years of trial and error, searching for help, knocking on every door.

On one particularly difficult day, I clearly remember looking to the sky and asking (begging) the universe to please send help.

Fifteen minutes later a call came from a kind woman I had never met. She lived about 600 miles away. A year earlier I had responded to her letter in a parents' forum in a magazine. She explained that she had since found help with a practitioner at the Hahnemann Clinic for Heilkunst and wanted to share with me. From that moment on lives were forever changed.

Today Matt is thirteen years old. Not only is he healthy, he is an extremely happy boy. He has grown four inches this year. He no longer suffers with *any* of his chronic ailments. Rarely does he even get a head cold. I honestly couldn't say when we last had antibiotics in our house.

Academically he still has many challenges ahead of him but he takes them on enthusiastically. Today he has a skip in his step rather than a limp. I can't imagine where we would be today if it were not for my practitioner and Heilkunst. The sparkle in Matt's eyes is a direct result of that knowledge and kindness. For that we are forever grateful."

3| What is Disease?

How do we know what a disease is, and how do we identify (diagnose) a particular disease when it occurs? Earlier we stated that disease was not simply an imbalance. Disease *produces* "dis-ease," but it is more than that. It is a form of impregnation of your generative power by a foreign influence that can only be removed (cured) by the use of medicines according to the natural law of similars.

Nature cures disease by the application of a similar disease. This is based on close observation of nature and cases of spontaneous cure in the medical literature. It is confirmed by centuries of clinical practice.

This was known by the ancients, but forgotten. It is even mentioned in Scripture.[2]

The law of opposites, used (mostly unconsciously) by conventional medicine, can only suppress symptoms. The painkiller may suppress a headache, but it does not cure the reason you have the headache. Conventional medicine is often rightly termed a "disease-management" system.

What we find masquerading as diagnosis in conventional medicine is basically a *description* of an arbitrary condition based on the visible, physical evidence caused by the counteraction of the sustentive power of our life force, and is not a true diagnosis of the underlying disease(s). The tip-off these days is that most new "diseases" are termed syndromes (Chronic Fatigue Syndrome, Acquired Immune Deficiency Syndrome, Sudden Acute Respiratory Syndrome) or disorders (Attention Deficit Disorder, Oppositional Defiant Disorder, etc.).

Let's imagine a physician comes across certain people with the same prominent physical symptom, such as painful swelling of the joints. He

---

[2] Mark 3:23 And he called them unto him, and said unto them in parables, How can Satan cast out Satan?
Mark 3:24 And if a kingdom be divided against itself, that kingdom cannot stand.
Mark 3:25 And if a house be divided against itself, that house cannot stand.
Mark 3:26 And if Satan rise up against himself, and be divided, he cannot stand, but hath an end.

takes this particular symptom or sign and gives it a name, drawing from Latin or Greek by tradition, and labels it "arthritis," thereby giving it a semblance of authority or reality it might not have on its own – arthritis just *means* inflammation of the joints, which sounds better than simply telling the patient, "You have inflammation of the joints."

Naming is fine, but does not in any way help in finding the *cause* of the condition. There usually are many theories, but no clear cause(s). That's because arthritis is a condition that is produced by one or more underlying diseases, and each patient will have a different disease, or series of diseases, that have caused that particular case of arthritis.

In one person it might be inherited, in another it might be due to chemical exposure, in another from deep or prolonged emotional shock. And in some cases, it might have nothing to do with disease proper, but is brought about by poor diet and nutrition, in which case you should properly apply the law of opposites, namely better diet and nutrition.

The medical world, whether conventional or alternative/ complementary, seems to run largely on these arbitrary conditions and false disease names rather than on a *true* understanding of disease. Name any product out there, or any therapy or treatment modality, and you will find cases of seemingly miraculous cures for arthritis. Yet, you will find at least ten cases *not* helped by that product or therapy for every one helped. How can this be? Because of the failure to understand what disease *really* is and how to distinguish disease from imbalance.

Imagine that we have ten people suffering from stomach (peptic) ulcers. They are all told first to simply drink more water (75% of people are chronically dehydrated and stomach ulcers are one result). After a few days one person has a dramatic and immediate recovery (and there are real cases of precisely this occurring). The others notice no, or only a slight, improvement.

The remaining nine are now told to eat a special diet. Two drop out of the program, their symptoms gone.

Next, we go to some form of energy balancing (acupuncture, shiatsu, Reiki) or exercise to relieve stress and tone the body – another two people leave, happy.

The others are growing frustrated as they see little or no improvement compared to their lucky counterparts. Why don't *they* get better, they ask? Well, their particular cause or sequence of causes has not yet been addressed. So far, we've been looking at imbalances (regimen and the law of opposites).

Next, we look to see if there are any identifiable diseases, such as emotional shocks, physical traumas, or inherited factors that must be addressed with medicine according to the law of similars. One person might have had the ulcer since losing his life partner or his job. Another may have been on drugs, one of the side-effects being a stomach ulcer from over-acidity. A third has had the ulcer after eating contaminated meat or fish while on a trip abroad.

Each of these causes is eventually addressed with the proper remedies used according to the law of similars and they, too, can be discharged from the group. Eventually, all are treated, but using different treatments and for different periods of time depending on the circumstances of their case. It may also be that, given the lack of perfectibility in human knowledge, that one case remains, the cause of the problem remaining a mystery – for now.

What can generate disease?

- toxins (chemicals, drugs, pollution, vaccinations)
- physical traumas (concussions, broken bones, deep wounds, injections)
- emotional shocks (suppressed grief, fear, shame, anger, etc.)
- infectious microbes (cholera, flu, typhoid, tuberculosis, etc.)
- inherited diseases and predispositions (more on this later)
- false beliefs about the world (illusions, delusions) – again, more about this later as it requires some explanation

If you have any of these they can potentially produce, on their own or in combination, almost any condition imaginable. Conventional medicine simply looks at the visible results, picks the most common symptom and gives it a name, presuming thereby to have identified a disease. If there is any treatment at all, it's really designed to manage the symptoms because there can be no true cure for an arbitrary condition.

As an example, we had a woman ask us to treat her daughter's urinary incontinence. We asked what the conventional diagnosis had been and she said, "exercise-induced incontinence." Apparently they hadn't found a Latin or Greek term for this yet! We asked what they had suggested as treatment, and she answered, "Nothing."

We then asked the young teen what sports she played, and she gave us a long list. We asked her if the incontinence happened during all of the activities and she said no, it only happened during karate class. We suggested that they had gotten the "diagnosis" wrong, and that it should have been more correctly termed "karate-induced incontinence!"

On further questioning, it turned out that young lady felt unfairly dealt with by her instructor and had a degree of suppressed anger. We gave her the appropriate medicine to remove the blockage to her healthy functioning caused by her suppressed anger and the condition went away. There never had been any "exercise-induced incontinence," only a disease caused by suppressed emotions, in this case anger.

In another case, a woman came into our office in tears because the doctors had told her she would have to learn to live with her chronic arthritic pain. She was told she could take aspirin (which didn't really help her pain and caused stomach problems), move to a dry climate or suffer until it became so bad that powerful painkillers would be prescribed. Needless to say, she didn't like any of the options she was offered by the rheumatologist despite his impressive degrees and many years of study.

We told her in all seriousness that we had no cure for "arthritis," but that we could remove (cure) the diseases causing it. We were eventually able to remove her arthritic condition, though it took some time due to the many diseases involved in this case, as it is for so many suffering with this condition.

Heilkunst is a system of medicine that provides a *true* identification (diagnosis) of disease, because as soon as you have identified the disease, the curative remedy is automatically known (it is disclosive, not just descriptive). Or, in some cases where the remedy is known through the symptoms alone, the nature of the disease is then known. The art lies in the skill of diagnosis, and there are many ways to make this relatively easy to do.

Two Types of Disease

The founder of Heilkunst, Dr. Samuel Hahnemann, discovered that there are two types of disease: diseases that are constant in nature and diseases that are variable.

The constant diseases, which we call tonic diseases, are those that always show up in the same manner, such as measles or chickenpox. Physical and emotional shocks also form tonic diseases – a contusion (bruise) is always the same, as is a concussion, and a shock related to the death of a loved one is equally constant in nature.

PATHIC DISEASE

Finally, we also have constant diseases caused by chemical toxins, including drugs. These diseases are hidden under the term "side-effects," which simply means that they are not the effects the chemical manufacturers want, but they are disease-effects nonetheless. The wonderful thing is that since the disease remains constant in nature, the medicine to cure the disease is also constant.

However, these tonic diseases can give rise to other diseases, which will depend on the time and circumstances of the case. These cannot be predicted or treated by knowing the cause (which is the tonic disease). You can only treat them by taking the symptoms produced and then matching this disease picture with the picture produced by a medicine.

We call these "pathic" diseases, from the Greek word "pathos," which means "suffering." The good news is that by treating for the tonic diseases, many of the pathic diseases are destroyed too, though occasionally a pathic disease will remain that will then need to be identified and removed.

Let's take a simple case of a child exposed to chickenpox who then comes down with the characteristic symptoms of the disease. Knowing it is chickenpox, we can give the child the specific medicine for chickenpox, which happens to be a highly diluted and potentized medicine made from the chickenpox virus (this *is* a disease-causing microbe, after all!). There is no longer any virus left in the remedy, but only the energetic vibration of the virus, and this is enough because the life force of the patient acts as if it was being given the actual virus.

According to the natural law of similar resonance the medicine meets the disease and, because two similar energetic patterns cannot exist in the same place, they destroy each other. The child may recover right away or, in a more extreme case, there may be some symptoms that linger. We then analyze any remaining symptoms and find a remedy that has the same symptom picture to remove the remaining pathic disease.

Provings

To find disease pictures or images we give healthy volunteers a highly diluted and dynamized substance (remedy) and then record what symptoms they produce. We call these tests *provings*. Remember, each substance has a potential effect on our life force. Since the substance is really in an energetic form it cannot create any lasting ill-effects on the healthy person.

You have probably carried out a proving, inadvertently, when you cut an onion – you get burning, watery eyes and an itchy, runny nose. These are symptoms similar to some allergic reactions, particularly hay fever, and the remedy potentized from a red onion (*Allium cepa*) is well-known for its remediation of allergy symptoms that are similar to those produced when cutting an onion.

The Law of Similars

The law of similars works everywhere in disease. You may have heard of its use in frostbite, where you are advised to use snow to gradually unfreeze the frozen part. To use heat (the law of opposites) would result in tissue damage.

It works equally well in the case of burns though we are taught, strangely enough, *not* to use it. Next time you have a burn try the law of similars. When you use cold, you get instant relief, but as soon as you remove the cold source, it starts to hurt badly and you can get long-lasting scars.

When you slowly re-expose the burn to heat (a similar, but not as intense as the heat that caused the burn) you will notice an immediate increase in discomfort, followed very quickly by a resolution of the pain and the quick recovery of the skin.

One of us recently spilled scalding hot tea water over his arm in a restaurant. We didn't have remedies with us, but remembered the law of similars and took the still quite warm mug and placed it against the burned arm for as long as could be tolerated, several times. Within a minute, the pain was gone and within about 30 minutes the angry red burn had disappeared.

The key, of course, is to remember the term "similar." If you use the same heat as caused the burn in the first place, you only get more of a burn. So, you have to use something less hot, but similar. It works!

Years ago, we encountered a blacksmith who explained how he treated burns, of which he had received many. He would put his burned part as close to the fire as he could stand. He stated that this helped it heal quickly and left no scarring. His arms were indeed devoid of scars. People were impressed, but no one understood why, as this went against the "official" advice.

We are also told to use cold packs when we have inflammation (swelling), like when we have a serious sprain or strain, but the law of similars would demand heat. Strangely enough this is what we do when we lightly strain our muscles, but when there is visible swelling it seems that conventional medicine doesn't trust the body's healing power and tries to suppress the evidence. Inflammation and heat is the way the body heals.

Alex's Story

Alex's case involved severe dysfunction coupled with a strong sensitivity to medicines. At the time of starting treatment with us, Alex had been diagnosed with several labels – Pervasive Developmental Disorder and Atypical Autism, in addition to various physical ailments.

According to his mother, his expression was very limited and he could not pay attention for more than a few seconds. He had no play skills and was having trouble learning and using language. On the other hand, there was no self-abusive or violent behavior.

He came with an extensive medical history from his birth, when his very low WBC count led to five days of intravenous antibiotics due to a fever on the second day of life. He was a large baby and needed to be suctioned at birth (often a sign of deeper inherited problems). The pushing stage of labor lasted two hours and his heart rate dropped during that time. Later, he seemed to have a pattern of receiving a shock and then falling back in terms of development and overall health because of it.

Alex's case is a very good example of autistic children whose problems lie not so much in the actual shocks, although they do destabilize and worsen the condition, but in the fact that they are born with severe weaknesses that strongly predispose them to being overwhelmed by any shock, making them hypersensitive and highly unstable.

The removal of the vaccination and drug shocks over the first year led to little apparent improvement, although he had some healing reactions as his body attempted to remove the heavy toxic load caused by the shocks. Changes were subtle and gradual.

We then began treating for the inherited weaknesses (chronic miasms), perhaps the most significant aspect of Heilkunst. Right from the start, the improvements became more noticeable. As Alex's mother stated: "This is the first time we feel that this is the right thing."

With one of the chronic miasms, Sycosis, there was a particular improvement – more interaction, happier, seeking out children to play with, using language more and communicating better, looking at books. His therapists also noticed a distinct improvement. Whereas this time of year was usually a difficult time for him, the Fall of 2000 proved to be easier than in the past. Where his fevers used to be continual, he had only a few days each month of fevers. His overall health continued to improve throughout the winter.

During the Fall of 2000, we also began a second round of treatments for the inherited diseases (chronic miasms). Again, the greatest improvement came with the treatment for Sycosis in April of 2001. And with the treatment at a deeper level for what is called the Syphilitic miasm, there was strong healing reaction, but also noticeable advances in receptive language.

Suddenly, some obsessive behavior emerged – wanting to sprinkle or pour water everywhere, not sleeping, fear of the dark, anxiety – all signs of a deeper realm we have termed the Chthonic (Greek word for earth) realm. This relates to the issue of fear, which is where much of the predisposition to autism resides because it provides the extreme sensitivity and predisposition to being destabilized by any shock or stress. A specific remedy helped to remove this compulsive behavior.

At one point, he suddenly developed a "malicious intent," acting destructively intentionally, which is a characteristic sign of the chronic miasm we term Tuberculosis. With the treatment, this behavior disappeared. Because of the deeper, more profound nature of the miasms at a higher level of treatment (in terms of potency or energy), it can take longer for the system to adjust to the stimulus and to restore health after the particular disease has been removed at the deeper level.

By the Spring of 2002, we were part of thc way through the second level of treatment of the miasms, when we received an emergency call from Alex's mother. He was acting "out of control," stripping naked, picking at his skin, stripping wallpaper and urinating and defecating on the floor. This was another emergence of the Chthonic realm, and was

Healing Reactions (Aggravations)

dealt with by another specific remedy for the disease state causing this behavior.

With the treatment for the Syphilitic miasm, Alex went through a difficult several months when things appeared to be regressing, particularly regarding his gastro-intestinal symptoms. Various dietary changes at this point helped considerably. He also required some treatment with Prednisone.

We continued on into the third level of treatment of the chronic miasms, and things started to improve. Alex's behavior was much better, his language skills grew, including the spontaneous use of words. Part of the improvement was due to the use of a new potency level, the LM or Q-scale, which seems to complement the traditional C-scale and can, in some cases, moderate the healing reactions.

A fourth round of treatment of the miasms began in the Fall of 2003. Again, there were various healing reactions with certain improvements. By the winter of 2004, Alex was doing "very well." And again, when the Syphilitic miasm approached he had stronger healing reactions, though continued gradual improvements.

Clearly, this has not been an easy case, and there will need to be further treatment to see what more improvement can be obtained. Alex has perhaps come to us as a teacher, helping us to learn more about autism, its depth and extent, and forcing us to extend the limits of our knowledge and therapeutics so that we can better help others. We have found that each child has contributed to our learning and to the greater effectiveness of the treatment that we can offer children trapped in the autistic condition.

Parent's Comments

I began with Heilkunst treatment in 1999, about four and a half years ago to try to improve the health of both my sons. Alex, who is now 10 years old, is profoundly autistic. He also has had terrible medical issues his entire life including immune suppression, colitis, cryptitis and lymphoid nodular hyperplasia. My younger son, Liam, is seven and is developing normally. But by the time he was one, he was covered in eczema most of the time and had developed asthma.

With Liam, homeopathic treatment using a sequential approach to his life traumas had an immediate and profound impact. Within six months or so, every sign of asthma had disappeared, never to return. It took another few years, but he's now also able to tolerate dairy and soy with no problems. He's also had no eczema for over a year.

Alex, being so much more profoundly ill, has been a much harder nut to crack. However, I say without any doubts that sequential trauma treatment has helped him. At this point, Alex's colitis is in complete remission and his immune system is functioning well enough to have him off the gamma globulin IVs we relied upon to keep him alive the previous seven years. In addition to the help he received from his treatment with the Hahnemann Clinic, he also benefited greatly from a diet we put him on a year ago. Certainly, the sequential trauma treatment in conjunction with other measures, such as diet, works very well, as they all support each other.

When trying to describe homeopathic treatment to someone unfamiliar with it – and the effects it has had on Alex – I go back to my personal favorite story. Several years ago, Alex was climbing everything in the house. What really had us scared was that he'd climb on and over the railing surrounding the hallway of our upstairs, hanging a story above the slate floor of our foyer. I called my Heilkünstler, desperate, because I truly feared for Alex's life. I was shipped what we affectionately have named, "Essence of Tarantula." Within 24 hours of the first drop, Alex stopped climbing and has never done anything remotely like that since.

If I had to describe exactly what each remedy seems to have done for Alex, I'd have to say that millimeter by millimeter, it has pushed him toward a greater state of physical health. While we haven't yet seen the tremendous language and cognitive gains that many of my friends with autistic children have, each time Alex comes out of a healing reaction, it's as though there's a tiny bit more clarity in his eyes… like we've managed to scoop one more teaspoon of water out of the bucket of his autism.

I trust the healing properties of homeopathy so much that I have strongly recommended it to many, many families with autistic children. Every one of them has seen tremendous benefits almost immediately. Alex's disease state, which is so incredibly deep-rooted, could not possibly have altered quickly. It's been four and a half years of a slow, but perceptible, change. As his health is now so much more improved, however, I fully hope and expect that future treatments will demonstrate the benefits I know they are capable of doing.

4| The Three Realms of Medicine

Any true system of medicine has three realms or divisions:

- Therapeutic regimen (diet, nutrition, lifestyle) – restoration of balance when the state of health is temporarily disturbed
- Therapeutic medicine proper – cure of disease
- Therapeutic education – providing the meaning for one's journey through life

We'd like to give you an outline of each of these in Heilkunst.

Therapeutic Regimen

There is a lot of advice out there about what to do and what not to do to remain healthy. Who should we believe?

First, it is important to determine jurisdiction. In human law, the issue of jurisdiction is the first thing considered. If you live in one state or province, the laws of another state or province don't apply to you. If you have committed an offence under federal law, then only federal courts and judges have jurisdiction over the case.

If you are a practitioner, you are the detective, arresting officer, prosecutor, judge, jury and bailiff all rolled into one. You have to determine if you have jurisdiction over the case (does it fall within your area of competence?) before you can act. You also have to decide in which court the case is to be tried (treated).

If it is a case of simple imbalance (not drinking enough water, for example, or not getting enough exercise), then you can't take it to Medical Court; it has to be tried in Regimenal Court.

Regimen is the realm of imbalance, or illness that is simply due to a lack or excess of something. It is easily corrected because it has only disturbed the sustentive power of our living principle, the Dynamis. The natural law that applies here is the law of opposites.

If you determine that a patient has not been getting enough of the right kind of nutrients, for example, or has an energy imbalance, then the sentence of the court (diagnosis) is clear. The patient must, to regain health, start eating the right nutrients or have the energy imbalance corrected. To *not* do so would be contempt of court (in this case an offense against natural law). The only punishment meted out in the case of a failure to follow the sentence of the court is one that you inflict on yourself – continued ill-health.

How do you tell what are the right kind of nutrients for a person or the best way to correct an energy imbalance? Heilkunst provides the principles that tell you what is right for your type or for your condition.

For example, if you are the product of a difficult birth, then the use of one of several manipulative methods to correct the distortion in the cranium and spine, such as osteopathy, cranio-sacral therapy or chiropractic, is warranted. If you are a particular blood type, have a particular dominant endocrine gland and have a certain metabolic type (all of which are easily determined) then the particular foods, supplements and exercise that are right for you will easily be known.

Therapeutic Medicine

If, however, you have acquired a disease the problem will not be fixed by any judgment from the Regimenal Court. Disease involves an impingement or damage to the generative power that can only be corrected by the application of the law of similars. No amount of right diet or energy work will remove the fact that you have a disease. Regimen can make you feel better and stronger, but the disease will continue to grow.

We recall a case where a patient found relief from her symptoms through various regimenal measures provided by a naturopath. She found, however, that the symptoms eventually came back and that she then felt worse than before. Why, she wanted to know, did this happen?

Disease needs to be prosecuted in front of a judge that has jurisdiction over the natural law of similars. Then, after the proper trial, the right sentence can be pronounced and the guilty properly dealt with. In the case of medicine it is not the fault of the patient, as it is in regimen. The guilty party is the disease, which must be identified and then removed with the proper remedy/medicine.

If a headache is caused by a concussion from a fall, then it *can only* and *must be* removed by the application of a medicine chosen on the basis of the law of similars. In this case it must be a medicine that has the power to cause, in a healthy person, the same symptoms of a concussion, even though that person has not had a concussion (it's *as if* they had – the law of similars). Again, the judgment of the court of medicine *can* be ignored, the patient can elect not to treat the disease, but the result is simply more suffering as the diseases and shocks accumulate.

Therapeutic Education

Much of our ill health and disease arises from ignorance. Since we cannot abide a pure state of ignorance, we have to fill in the vacuum of knowledge with belief. If the belief is understood as a temporary and not necessarily a true explanation of reality, we have a hypothesis and we have science.

If a belief is treated as being true, even in the face of evidence to the contrary, and any challenge of the belief is met with emotional reaction or attacks on the messenger, we have superstition and false belief.

False belief eventually leads to false thinking, which in turn leads to customs and traditions. These, then, are the means to inculcate subsequent generations in the false belief. It is a self-perpetuating system, and the only remedy here is truth.

DE-GENERATIVE DISEASE

This is a tricky issue, as we are all subject to error. However, this is not to say that we cannot know truth. Truth comes from our deeper, inner knowing, from the realm of cosmic wisdom that we were given at birth. Truth is more a matter of recognition than of learning something new. A teacher is a guide to our own discovery of this inner wisdom and helps us to bring it into our consciousness so that it doesn't just remain as a feeling or "gut instinct."

Science is now talking about the discovery of a brain that is more complex and has more nerve endings than our brain mind. This other brain is situated in our solar plexus or gut, and is our body mind.

When we *know* something we feel a sense of recognition of self and connection to the universe that gives us peace of mind. We are *not* upset when this knowing is challenged, for our knowing is not a belief, uncertain and open to doubt. We do not have to have others agree with it, as truth is not a matter of how many people support it. Even if no one agrees with us, it remains the truth.

We've all had "ah-ha!" moments, those "eureka" experiences when we "got" something, or when a solution to a problem presented itself to us. This is the wellspring of all creativity. Science is founded by geniuses, who are geniuses precisely because they can, more than most of us, tap into this deep, inner knowing of all things and then present it to the world as a gift in the form of a new insight or a new machine or device to make life easier (and more complicated, too!).

We *all* have this capacity for genius, except that we either don't listen to it, or we don't do anything specific with it. But we can develop our ability to tap into this capacity. Disease shuts us off from this ability, particularly chronic disease, which is why we tend to call it "*de*-generative," because it weakens our generative or creative power.

Health in terms of freedom from chronic disease is a pre-condition for the constructive and rational use of our inner genius. Most natural genius, if not in a healthy person, tends to be destructive (mad scientist) or self-destructive (mad artist). Like the energy of an exuberant and active child, it needs to be channeled into constructive pursuits.

Thus, a large part of becoming healthy, and of any system that works to bring a person to health, must be the ability to develop our organs of inner knowledge and the ability to make sense of this new world. We have to live in this world of matter and the external senses, but we also need to integrate our *inner* knowing with our *outer* world, which is *true* science.

Bridging the Duality

This is precisely what Heilkunst does – it brings us into contact with our inner self through a journey into our past traumas, to retrieve and bring into the whole the parts of our soul that have been left stranded in time (perhaps the time, for example, at age eight when you had a severe emotional shock, or at two months when you had your first vaccination). In a sense, you *can* travel back into time. While your physical body remains behind, your energetic and soul bodies can actually time travel, and you can heal the accumulated shocks and traumas of your past.

Part of this past that we have to overcome and transform comes from events in this lifetime, but it is clear that part of it comes in with us when we are born. We definitely know that there is a genetic inheritance of conditions, even diseases such as syphilis or TB. This is on the natural, or earth, side of our being, the side of the Dynamis.

There is also growing evidence that we have a different kind of inheritance, one that comes from the side of Spirit (Spiritus). This is the origin of many of our spiritual diseases, involving ignorance and false beliefs. Any *true* medical system has to address both the natural and the spiritual diseases, which Heilkunst does.

Geoffrey's Story

Geoffrey, age six, has been treated at the time of this writing for just over seven months. His parents have had him on a strong program of supplements and dietary restrictions, which had provided some benefits.

From the initial sequential treatment to remove the various shocks during his short lifetime, he showed increased confidence or expression, greater assertion and some spontaneous language, and seemed stronger in his overall health. This provides, as in other cases, a clear illustration of the value not only of what we term regimenal measures, which provide a greater degree of balance but do not remove the underlying causes, but also of medicine proper, according to natural laws, that actually work to eliminate these causes.

To use chelation therapy, for example, to remove high levels of heavy metals like mercury and many others, does not remove the *cause* of these high levels. Although there is mercury in many of the childhood vaccinations, even this does not explain the actual level of mercury in many autistic children, much less that of lead or cadmium, which is not generally expected in vaccine material.

After the second month, he showed increased use of language. By the fourth month his mother stated he was "doing great," had become more talkative and adventuresome, with big jumps in comprehension and language skills after treatment for a fall and cut to his head.

We also treated with a remedy to try to stabilize his gut and found that his slapping activity decreased markedly. He now followed directions better, recounted what was happening on TV without any prompting, showed a greater interest in his surroundings and became more self-directed.

At his last consultation to date, his mother indicated that he experienced a "huge jump" in his abilities for no apparent reason, other than the remedies for the last trauma treated, which had been the MMR vaccination. The removal of this trauma had also allowed his system to get rid of much of his heavy metal toxicity. He is now talking more, using more imaginative play, and has, in his mother's words, "crossed another threshold."

Parent's Comments

The following is a précis of our journey to date with Geoffrey as we attempt to heal his autistic condition.

Our son Geoffrey is marvelous and we love him unconditionally as we do his younger sister, Olivia. Geoffrey was diagnosed with autistic spectrum disorder of a severe nature on June 11, 2002 at 3:00 in the afternoon. He was four-and-a-half years old. When Geoffrey was six months old he would sometimes stare at lights and not turn his head when we called his name. At eight months we started getting "early intervention" because he had low muscle tone.

During the next three and half years Geoffrey saw an endocrinologist three times, a neurologist two times, a psychologist two times, a geneticist twice. He had an EEG, an EKG, an abdominal ultrasound, a CAT scan and an MRI (which required a general anesthesia). We saw a developmental pediatrician who informed us our son was not autistic but would likely begin seizuring soon due to a rare condition (I had already researched this and ruled it out).

We spent a lot of time trying very hard to find out what was causing our sons apparent confusion in this world. Within two months of Geoffrey's diagnosis we had removed all gluten and casein from his diet. Within four months we had attended our first conference on biomedical interventions in ASD (DAN! movement). Within a year we had begun chelation therapy to remove heavy metals we had found using specific challenge testing.

After Geoffrey was diagnosed I began meeting other parents who were also attempting to heal their children either through biomedical interventions or homeopathy or both. I met one particular mother who had been very impressed with the language she had seen in her son after seeing a homeopath. My husband and I were quite skeptical of homeopathy as a treatment modality. I did say that I would consider homeopathy only after I had exhausted all of the biochemical options, and the reason I gave was that I knew very little about homeopathy and did not think I could understand it, and if I could not understand a treatment modality then I could not, in good conscience, apply that therapy to my son.

One year after carefully venturing into biomedical interventions we went to the United States to visit a very well respected DAN! (biomedical) doctor. She is very careful, thoughtful and respectful of the healing process in our children. She also incorporates a type of energy medicine into her practice, which was not homeopathy. We respected this doctor's approach and accessed the energy medicine she had to offer, and saw positive changes in Geoffrey. He is generally very shy and quiet and he began to express himself and assert himself.

When we came home to Canada I felt somehow that we were missing something important in our perspective on healing. We were looking at healing from the science we knew, not the science we did not know. We were looking at healing at the cellular level instead of healing at a less tangible, but perhaps more important level, that of the energy of the whole body. We decided to learn as much as we could about homeopathy, in other words to open our minds and research how this healing modality is supposed to work.

We found the study of homeopathy to be fascinating and mind-expanding. One particular statement stays with me, and that was that North American evidence-based medicine is one of the few approaches in the world that does not take into account an energy or vital force as a component of healing. As a result of our readings we decided to pursue homeopathy, and in particular sequential homeopathy. As soon as we made our decision I felt that we had changed our healing approach from linear to circular in nature.

My son, our four-year-old daughter and myself have been taking sequential homeopathic remedies (which I admit are very much easier to administer than all our biomedical supplements) for seven months now. The following are some of the notes I have made after treatments on Geoffrey.

1) Five days post introduction of the basic dropper bottle - increase in confidence, trying to express himself using different words than the usual.
2) After treatment for yeast overgrowth - great weekend, lots of language, "Hey Olivia this is the big boy's store," (aka Canadian Tire) and so proud to tell her this as she was in the store with him. Trying new physical positions (low motor tone, so generally very cautious).
3) After stronger yeast treatment - had clear discharge from nose and rash on cheeks and very, very tired in therapy (head on desk). Clear discharge changed to thick mucopurulent discharge for about seven days.
4) After new dropper bottle (stronger) very talkative, took his shirt and undershirt off himself (which he doesn't ever do), threw rocks in the planter, then urinated in the planter (we thought all this was great because he was interested in experimenting with his environment), also more emotional of late, cries more easily.
5) Ten days after above - he gave each of us a hug… awesome!!!!
6) Ten days plus after Varicella (chickenpox) - huge jump in language and comprehension, follows directions better, not so foggy, telling us what's happening on TV, kicking rocks into the drain like a regular little six-year-old boy would, pulling up plants from planters and pouring out people's coffees. Again we thought this was great as it was all new.
7) After MMR, very, very tired, seems foggier again and very sensitive to tone in my voice; also flapping a lot. He was in the bath and I just shifted him over and he started to cry, then he said, "Can I have some sage and lemongrass scrub to make me feel better"!!!!!

After about six months of therapy we became aware that apart from the variations in behavior and language we would see connected to each powder or dropper bottle, that overall Geoffrey seemed to be so much happier with his state of being. He would laugh and smile so much more; his face held much more expression and his eyes now twinkled. He is beginning to open his windows to let us in.

My husband and I are both doctors. He is a dentist and I am a veterinarian. We are truly grateful for the change in perspective that our son has brought us to. We are perhaps not evolved enough to rely entirely on homeopathy to heal our son and therefore continue to use chelation therapy, supplements, behavioral therapies and far-infrared saunas. We absolutely feel that sequential homeopathy is addressing healing at a level that cannot be reached using biomedical interventions. And so the journey continues… filled with love, faith, hope and the never-ending quest for understanding.

5| The Meaning of Disease and Illness

This brings us to a very difficult question, namely *why* do we get sick or, more commonly asked, "Why do bad things happen to good people?"

The answer is partly given in those accounts by remarkable people who tell of their struggle with a serious illness or disease and how it has altered their life for the better. It comes from the changed lives people lead after a near-death experience. Illness and disease are adversaries that we have been given to test ourselves against so that we may have the opportunity to become who we were meant to be, or given the potential to be, by our Creator.

Disease has a profound meaning *if* we are open to receiving it. While no one would wish an illness or disease on anyone, we cannot deny that disease has the power to alter our lives. We may say that we like or dislike something or that it is either pleasant or unpleasant, but we cannot really say that something is "bad" or "good" in a moralistic way, for that is to judge, which is the province of a higher power than us.

If we look back on our lives we often have to acknowledge that the experiences that were the most challenging and unpleasant were also the ones that changed us the most, for the better. As our parents often would say, adversity builds character, or "In every adversity is the seed of an equal or greater benefit." Or some parents would say that what doesn't kill us makes us stronger!

As humans we have a tendency to remain static, to desire only one side of things, usually the sweet side. We don't like the bitter, but as any herbalist will tell you, too much sweet disturbs the digestion – a little touch of bitter herbs will set things right again.

Polarity

The world is built around polarities. We have both a spirit and a dynamic pole within us. We have both a generative and a sustentive power within our Dynamis or Life Force. We cannot know light unless we also know dark. Of course, light will always overcome dark, but to be light it has to have the dark. Indeed, as the German scientist Goethe showed us, and as any artist knows (and contrary to what Newton taught), color emerges out of the interplay of light and dark.

In fact, the sky is blue because that is the color produced when pure light (sunlight) is seen against a pure dark background (space). Also, the colors in the morning sky (blue spectrum) are produced when the light meets the dark and the colors of the sunset are produced when the dark comes to meet the light (red spectrum).

We cannot know health without knowing illness or disease. Illness and disease are like confinements or prisons. They restrict our freedom as human beings. We cannot really be free if we have not first known imprisonment, and we cannot be truly free unless we overcome that struggle. Others can help us, but we need to do it for ourselves. The fight against illness and disease is a very personal struggle, one that is very lonely, but one that has the ability also to set us free spiritually.

Thus, it is hard to say that disease is "bad" in a moral sense. It is simply an adversary, which is the meaning of the Hebrew term "Satan" in scripture. We can and *must* struggle against illness and disease. That is our responsibility, for it is also the path to freedom as human beings.

Freedom means having a sense of inner joy and calm that comes from knowing ourselves, and from knowing that the world and its experiences are not punishments or rewards from capricious gods, but simply a gigantic stage for finding ourselves. We learn to be free of fear and learn to love ourselves and the world with all its imperfections. And we learn to trust that all of it is for our spiritual journey, but that we *can* make changes by our own creative power.

In its deepest sense, we discover that the world around us is but a reflection of our state of mind or consciousness, and that if we change this state of mind, the world changes as well (the basis for the seemingly puzzling placebo effect).

Love is Letting Go...

We had a patient who complained that no one loved her and that everyone always abandoned her. She eventually discovered that she had a belief that no one could ever love her because she was not *worthy* of any love. When she became healthy enough to acknowledge this belief and overcame her fear of challenging it, she discovered that the world is indeed full of love. And she found a resonant intimate relationship with someone who reflected her unconditional love and acceptance of herself.

Previous lovers could never love her enough, because she could never trust their love so long as she believed that she was not worthy of *being* loved. Eventually, they left her and thus her belief was confirmed, a self-fulfilling prophecy. This only deepened her sense of failure and unworthiness.

Now, instead, she has a sense of trust in love and a sense that the world is built on love. She can see in the difficult passages the love of the universe pressing us to explore our inner selves and to come into our own power and light.

It's hard to tell someone who's suffering that this is a necessary part of life and that it actually has universal love behind it. However, from a spiritual perspective this is indeed the case. We achieve freedom when we understand that the energy that drives the universe of the Creator *is* love, and that all of it is neither good nor bad, but are experiences designed to help us unfold who we are.

Thus, it is not that bad things happen to good people, but that *things* happen to *people,* and we have to trust that there is a deeper spiritual purpose behind all events even if we cannot see what they might be, particularly through our pain. Hindsight is good for that!

The Role of Medicine

Medicine is a gift from the Creator that allows us to remove suffering much faster than might normally be the case, and also to tackle deep issues that we might not otherwise be strong enough to handle. Spiritual growth is like human growth. As we mature, we are given more and more responsibility along with our freedom. In our work we also undertake greater responsibility and challenges as we grow in our experience and abilities.

However, medicine must act according to natural law, otherwise it will lead to harm, no matter how much good it may appear to be doing. Of course in Heilkunst there *is* a place for surgery, antibiotics and chemical drugs, but they *must* be used within their jurisdiction, so their role is limited and severely restricted. To use them routinely and repeatedly, other than in severe emergencies where the life force is almost gone or is seriously threatened, is to harm. To use medicine outside natural law principles and jurisdiction is to suppress the spiritual path that each person has before them.

We must go to meet our suffering and then, with the aid of medicine acting lawfully, to transform it, and not hide from it or suppress it. If we follow natural and spiritual law, as is the case in Heilkunst, we achieve spiritual growth and true inner peace and knowing. We come to live fully in the world, yet to act according to the dictates of our deep, inner knowing and desire (or love). We live in unconditional love and follow that love where it resonates so that we experience deep fulfillment, a treasure and wealth that is beyond measure and that cannot be taken away by anyone.

The following comments were written by a patient who had come to see us two years ago and who had been on a long journey of suffering without any apparent end. At times she fell into despair, as she had not yet gained a sense of the purpose of her life and journey. There still remains much to be done for her to achieve greater health, but the difficult point of self-acceptance has been reached (grace) and what remains is the maturing into her self.

Thoughts:

I thought that I had to construct the answer like a jigsaw puzzle.
I discovered that the answer was there by deconstructing what I thought the puzzle was.

I thought I needed to tell the truth of each piece of my ego-self in order to fit them together.
I discovered that the truth was a whole, which revealed itself once I stepped back from the puzzle and saw that the ego-self wasn't real.

I thought that I needed to strive and struggle to get well, which involved a *lot* of very detailed study.
I discovered that while all that was going on, the real healing connection was being made higher up, and the dance of the lower mental stuff wasn't what was holding things together at all.

I thought I knew all these things ages ago, and I did on a certain superficial level of understanding. But I discovered these things internally as they finally began to come to life within me.

The struggling phase that came before the discovery phase seems optional to me now, in a certain sense. But it was only my doing the struggle so obtrusively, giving it a form so that I could see and understand it, that I could finally see it for what it really was. It was just a superficial structure, but I had to play it out until I was tired of playing with shadows.

I thought I was tired of it years ago, but if you identify with something, no matter how much it pains you, you can't let it go.

You complain and struggle to get free, but it's a Gordian knot that ties you even tighter the more you struggle.

Now I come to the turning point, realizing that the struggle is optional. This doesn't mean that I didn't have to do the work or go through what I did, only that the reason for doing it isn't the reason I believed.

I thought I was struggling to get free; I discovered I was struggling in order to come to the realization that I'm already free. And from that perspective, the struggle that I identified with before starts to fall away because my sense of self is somewhere else.

That's how I'm being released from the compulsion to struggle. That's how a person is transformed from an unconscious player with no freedom of choice, to a conscious and free person. Maybe we learn to discern the real from the unreal by our continued experience with these dark shadows. And life gives us plenty of ways to do that.

Now the story that I've been telling of the elements of my struggle becomes a story of shadows. It has no substance of its own in the truest sense. It's not to be mistaken for the story of a life, the deeper healing of the heart. Now I trust my authentic life unfolding out of the shadows from here on.

6| A Model for Autistic Conditions

Although each case is unique, they all consist of a series of similar factors that help to organize and simplify treatment. From our research and clinical experience, and from our understanding of disease, we can see the following model that lies behind the emergence, both in a single, specific case and generally, as a growing incidence in early infantile autism.

Inherited factors - the predisposition

Generally, there are seven archetypal chronic diseases (chronic miasms) that produce a myriad of symptoms in any given person. Most people are born with all of these chronic miasms to a greater or lesser degree. They generally lie dormant within us until they are activated by certain shocks.

Those children who become autistic generally will have one or both parents or grandparents that have certain behavioral traits indicative of one or more of the chronic miasms. Two of the miasms in particular, one that is derived from an original syphilitic infection and the other from an original case of gonorrhea (both somewhere in the family tree, even several generations back) are particularly strong.

People with autism can have a tendency to sensory disturbances, allergies, gastrointestinal problems, depression, obsessive compulsiveness, epilepsy, ADHD and strong anxiety, all of which are found strongly in the two chronic miasms mentioned above. Some of these same symptoms, in particular repetitive or compulsive behaviors, are often found in parents or grandparents.

The Triggers:

Vaccination

The main factor that acts to trigger the chronic miasms into action is frequent and multiple childhood vaccinations. The publication of an article by Dr. Andrew Wakefield and associates in a 2002 issue of *The Lancet* provided evidence of the role the MMR vaccine (measles, mumps, rubella) in causing autism.

However, it is not *just* the MMR, but *many* of the vaccinations that are the problem. Harris L. Coulter and Barbara Loe Fisher state, in *DPT: A Shot in the Dark* (1985), "The phenomenon of early infantile autism was first observed and discussed by physicians in the early 1940s, a few years after the pertussis vaccine became more widely used in the United States... The parallel to certain areas of pertussis vaccine damage is striking."
(p. 123).

The miasm sycosis, that derived from an original gonorrheal infection, at some point in the family history, is the origin of many allergic-like symptoms and conditions and is at the root of the strong reactions of some children to the viral content of the vaccine. This was first noticed by homeopaths in the 19th century (after the smallpox vaccine) and was named "vaccinosis" by J. Compton Burnett.

Mercury

Those with a syphilitic miasm are particularly sensitive to mercury and other heavy metals, which are found in most vaccinations. Mercury poisoning was first noticed in hat makers in London several centuries ago (hence the term "mad as a hatter"), and in more recent times became famous due to mercury poisoning in Minamata, Japan from mercury-contaminated fish.

Levels of mercury that might be considered safe by the public health "authorities" can produce extreme reactions in very sensitive children, and those with a strong syphilitic miasm in their background are born with this hypersensitive predisposition. Researchers in Japan have found that even very low levels of mercury (just ten parts per million in hair and umbilical cords), some five times *lower* than the so-called "safe" levels, will produce neurological damage and block the functioning of various senses (sight, hearing, smell, taste and touch).

Much of the information linking mercury in drugs and vaccines can be found at www.safeminds.org. Safe Minds (Sensible Action For Ending Mercury-Induced Neurological Disorders) is a non-profit parents' organization founded to investigate the continuing risks to infants and children from exposure to mercury from medical drugs and vaccines. Annex G provides a link to a video produced by the Faculty of Medicine of the University of Calgary, showing the effects of small doses of mercury on a brain motor neuron.

The syphilitic miasm is also at the origin of obsessive-compulsive, bi-polar and addictive behavior, as well as causing an inability in people to connect with the world around them. Many such people are highly creative, but often self-destructive.

Traumas - mental, emotional, physical

Each child will react differently to any given shock. In some cases one shock is sufficient to trigger the appearance of an autistic condition in a child, and in others it requires a series of shocks. What seems to be the most common trigger across the board are childhood vaccinations.

From our perspective, the concept of prevention through immunization is a sound one; indeed, the approach is based on the natural law of similars. However, from time immemorial, it has been known that the law of similars is very dangerous because it is *so* powerful in its action when the dose is *too large*, or still in its crude, material state.

It was not until the 18th Century that a way was found, through a process of dynamisation and potentisation (often referred to as a "homeopathic dose") to render the application of the curative law of similars entirely safe (*see Annex C on Homeopathic Pharmacy*). However, the crude viral doses used in conventional vaccinations (and children's vaccinations can be stronger than those for adults), the increasing number of children's vaccinations (some 30 or more within the first several years of a child's life), plus the emerging practice of combining several vaccines (often as many as five or six) into one injection, not to mention the cumulative effect of the various heavy metals (such as mercury) and chemicals in such vaccinations, is akin to playing with fire.

It's on the official record that conventional vaccinations can kill and seriously maim. In fact, when researchers want to *create* encephalitis in laboratory animals they inject them with the pertussis (whooping cough) vaccine.

It is equally well-known that vaccines stress the immune system. We consistently find that when a child is treated for a vaccination shock with the appropriate remedies, their health improves significantly, and the more they are treated for, the greater the improvement in health.

Less serious effects of vaccinations are earaches and "infections," frequent colds, strep throats, difficulty focusing and irritability, with more serious effects including allergic reactions, environmental sensitivities, cognitive delays and difficulties, hyperactivity, and varying degrees of behavioral problems, including autism. Other shocks to the system, though more in the nature of events that flow from the effects of the vaccinations, are antibiotics, anti-inflammatories and other drug interventions.

A common pattern we have seen in our clinic is for a child to develop normally for their first 6-12 months of life, with various health problems emerging after 4-6 months, during the time of the initial series of three DPTP/HI(b) vaccinations. These are then treated with drugs and antibiotics. The child may or may not seem to recover, but then the MMR vaccination at around 12-18 months seems to be a blow from which the child does *not* recover.

Parents will often identify a vaccination as the starting point of health problems, sensing that the health of their child has been compromised in a way that will not go away with time. Given the official stance on vaccinations (they are good and they do not harm), parental concerns are dismissed or ignored by authorities and doctors.

While in Canada children are still spared the Hepatitis B vaccination until around age 12 or 13, in the United States many states now require this vaccination within 24 hours of birth. Since the introduction of this requirement, cases of early infantile autism have sky-rocketed.

Of course, a given vaccination in and of itself is not sufficient to produce an autistic condition in a child; this requires inherited factors that allow the vaccination shock to severely destabilize the child. For this reason, we cannot say that early childhood vaccinations *alone* produce autism, but they are a significant factor or trigger in virtually *all* autistic cases we have seen.

7| A Treatment Approach

Any treatment of a complex condition like autism must have a systematic approach or map, otherwise one risks simply thrashing about in the labyrinth of disease, never finding the way out. As indicated, the main focus of treatment lies in the two realms of therapeutics:

- therapeutic regimen (law of opposites to treat imbalances), and
- therapeutic medicine proper (the use of the law of similars to remove disease).

The third realm, that of therapeutic education, is more directed at the parent (to aid in their comprehending the situation) than at the patient, often too young to understand this higher realm. This book and the resources mentioned herein are the beginning of this education.

In a deep sense, autistic children are guides to the beginning of stepping outside the box, the "matrix" or paradigm in which we have been living mostly unaware, and in a form of dream consciousness. They force use to confront reality and to learn painfully how to discern the meaning of life and our role in it. Where we were content to exist within a framework with little question, we are now forced to question much of what we once accepted.

In a very real sense, these children are here to show us how to become individuals, with a greater degree of consciousness about the world and our role in it. The traits that are identified in the book, *Indigo Children*, indicate the higher spiritual role that these individual spirits are to carry out:

- They have a strong sense of self-worth,
- They question authority and routine,
- They are highly creative,
- They respond to those who understand them, and withdraw from others (resonant relationship principle),
- They are free of manipulation by guilt,
- And they express their needs openly.

From a Heilkunst perspective, these are all qualities of a sovereign individual. It seems that we are shifting as a world to a deeper appreciation of higher values and our uniqueness, away from authority, tradition and materially-bound definitions of self. This requires a profound willingness to be more open and to know one's *true* self, to take full responsibility for one's actions and to live life according to an inner ethic rather than an outer morality.

Of course, this puts us into conflict with the material, one-sided, color-blind intellect that dominates our public world. To go counter to this authority-based system and to rely on one's own deep sense of what is right and wrong requires us to open ourselves to a higher power, to accept confusion and doubt, venturing into strange territory of the mind, soul and spirit.

It also requires us to act on the basis of love or resonance with that inner truth. That requires a lot of soul courage and opening of eyes and ears so that we can "see" that to which we would otherwise be blind, and "hear" that to which we would otherwise be deaf.

These children have come in some way to show us the way forward, to challenge the old patterns and to develop new ones based on the second industrial revolution in technology around the silica chip and its binary system (on/off). As a result of their openness of spirit, these children are more vulnerable to becoming destabilized by the improper use of that technology, particularly in the medical field, and particularly regarding interventionist and invasive methods such as ultrasound, drugs and vaccinations.

Vaccinations are particularly destabilizing because of their *known* ability to damage the general immune system from the shock of the injection of crude microbial material and various toxic chemicals directly into the bloodstream. The number of vaccinations in childhood has been growing rapidly over the years, from two or three vaccinations a few decades ago to 30+ in childhood now, and it is a recipe for disaster.

Regimen

To maintain health it is important to provide the right nutrients and to avoid toxic substances. There are also a variety of different therapies that can help alleviate many of the symptoms and behavioral issues of autistic children. Many of these are being explored by parents and different organizations and practitioners, and many will help improve the condition, but what remains is the problem of where to start and which therapy will help which child.

Because of the multiplicity of therapies out there, and the lack of an overall framework within which to order them, parents and caregivers are left to sort things out by themselves and to rely on trial and error. While Heilkunst itself has a long way to go to bring order in practical terms to the therapeutic confusion on the regimenal side, it has developed various principles to identify a sequence and hierarchy of therapies so that they can be better applied in any given case.

The key is to understand the essence of a therapy, namely what nugget of gold it brings to treatment that is not offered by any other therapy, and also which therapies are interchangeable. The problem is that each therapy is invented, often by chance or necessity, without any deeper understanding of the principles and natural laws at work. If it then attains some success, the therapist who uses this method easily falls prey to the "hammer" fallacy, namely that if all you have is a hammer, everything looks like a nail. Each therapy can claim to achieve an *effect* in a given case if enough energy and resources are applied, but this is not the same thing as removing a given obstacle to cure.

For example, if Vitamin C therapy has value, it is only for two reasons:

1. to remove any blockage to cure caused by a Vitamin C deficiency
2. to palliate any pain or discomfort.

In the first case, this is the essence of Vitamin C therapy. In the second case, this can only be justified on the temporary grounds of symptom relief pending a more effective removal of the *actual* cause using another therapy or medicine.

To pretend that the removal of symptoms by the use of mega-doses of Vitamin C will be an effective treatment (beyond that required to correct a deficiency) is to pretend what never was and never will be.

It is true that the level of the deficiency of Vitamin C will vary according to other factors. Initially, a patient under stress and with various other diseases and imbalances may have a high need for Vitamin C, but this level will decline as they are removed. If a person works only with Vitamin C therapy, massive doses will be needed to manage the case, but if other effective therapies and treatments are applied against other causes of the condition in the patient, much less Vitamin C will be required and eventually only to the point that is necessary for normal metabolic functioning.

Medicine

In true medicine the main focus is on the blockages that have penetrated the generative side of the life force, which *cannot* be removed by regimenal measures alone. While Vitamin C may alleviate inflammation caused by a vaccination shock, the shock itself can only be removed by a remedy that is given in a safe dose (diluted and energized) and according to the law of similars.

There is no iatrogenic effect, meaning disease-causing effect (often dismissed as "side-effects"), in this bio-energetic medicine. There *can* be healing reactions, which represent the effort of the sustentive side of the life force to restore balance once a particular disease has been removed.

There are all sorts of toxins that need to be eliminated and repairs that need to be made by a person's innate natural healer. This is accomplished by means of inflammation and discharges, which are often temporarily uncomfortable, but do not cause any lasting negative effects.

Such efforts at healing are often misinterpreted by the conventional medical system as simply a sign of disease and something that needs to be suppressed with painkillers or antibiotics. While such measures *usually* are counter-productive, in some cases they *can* provide some relief if used judiciously where the pain and discomfort is great.

The following is from an exchange between parents regarding the issue of the healing reaction on an on-line support group:

> *You bring up an important point about the relationship between negative reactions and regression. A negative reaction goes away - lasts for a few hours or days or even weeks. But it goes away. I wouldn't say that was regression. Regression would be, say, if my son lost a level of speech, or lost a physical skill or a social skill or the like. And that would be true only if it persisted for a long time, not just if one day he didn't do something because he was having a rough time with the reactions to the remedy.
>
> Now obviously, the real kicker here is how long is long. I mean as you live through it - one day can be a long time. But I would say that as far as detox is concerned, I didn't really see anything that lasted much past a week or two, and most things changed and were better and worse during that time. In fact, I don't recall any reaction to a specific detox that lasted longer than that detox itself. Basically the same is true of Sequential. [Referring to the part of Heilkunst where the diseases are removed in a sequential manner, observing a chronological a timeline of the patient's traumas.]
>
> And yet I would say that overall for my son, there was a significant difference between reactions to detox and to Sequential. With Sequential he had a very severe reaction to the first booster, which was DPT OPV (which I would

say was the first and crucial hit to his system). That booster was his second remedy.

The first was an antibiotic which he showed no more reaction to than the average detox at that point. After the 1M of that booster, my son went into severe negative reactions. He stayed there for more than a month, and he climbed out very slowly. Overall, he was like someone struggling all the time from that day in Aug of 98 until he cleared to the 10M for the first time - which was the chicken pox vaccination.

Then it was as if a lid or a heavy object had been removed. Then I really began to see emerging the enormous gains he was making. But most of the gains did not really come into full view until the last vaccination was cleared. Then he burst forth like the first flowers of spring - suddenly a whole new season began.

I think the way to judge a therapy is by its results. The negative reactions are not the results. They are what you must go through to get the results.

The results of Sequential - the timeline part [addressing the traumas chronologically] - are fantastic. I would do it again and recommend it to others even if it were 10 times as difficult as it was. The results are that good.

I hope that my son's case was unusually difficult, and that others will have an easier time of it. It wouldn't surprise me, if that is the way it turns out...

I hope my all too vivid descriptions of the negative reactions don't deter you. They weren't intended to do that. They were intended to arm you with the knowledge of what the very worst might look like. But you will know that even that worst resulted in enormous positive gains.

We are five months away from [the treatment of the] birth [trauma] with our older son (age 7) and I find that I am getting that anxious feeling again. I had wanted to jump over the OPV/Hep B booster for the holiday break and proceed to the original DPT vaccine, but was advised to do that booster first. It ended up being a good idea because we saw some nice changes in time for Christmas. This was after struggling most of December with colds and sore throats.

So anyway, I am pleased to announce that we had one of the best Christmases in about five years. My son enjoyed every one of his gifts.

In the past he would open a gift, put the wrapping paper on one side and the present on the other and look as though he could not wait for the torture to end. This year he stood in the living room and said “Santa.” We also heard him say “snowman” several times despite the fact that it was not a white Christmas. He opened each gift, labeled them and played with many. (Play is not usually his strong suit.)

I have noticed that the occasional food slips don’t make as big as a dent as they used to. I think he had one last night and it made for a restless night’s sleep, but by mid AM was over. I too want to do another food allergy screen of some sort, because I suspect that the old ones may have changed. If anyone can recommend a good one to ask for let me know. I also spoke to a naturopathic MD (my friend’s sister) recently and she said that some people are very close to developing a digestive enzyme. We exchanged e-mail addresses, so I hope to write her soon and find out more. This was the person who suggested that I try Seacure and it has really helped. People suspect that seacure works in the intestines.

At this time in the timeline we have seen a great improvement in behavior and social ability, although social still has very far to go. Cognitive has its ups and downs. The poops did also change and for the most part have stayed healthy since last summer when we went by the original MMR. I no longer consider him to fit the chronic diarrhea definition. I am really hoping for the language and learning to come in. As usual, time will tell.

Our 6 year old is nearing birth and doing pretty well. I would say that I am concerned with his auditory processing so I am trying to read up on the listening url's that you had posted not too long ago...

I think we should be into the miasms soon as he just sailed through the original DPT with no problems.

A Case Study

Actual cases are not proof of anything, because *all* approaches and therapies will have impressive successes. Heilkunst, however, is not so much a specific therapy or approach, but a framework of principles grounded in natural law that provides a scientific guide to effective treatment on a consistent basis *regardless* of the case at hand.

Actual examples can help, however, to illustrate how each case will be approached and what might be expected to happen. Of course, the details of each case will vary as the arbitrary label of autism hides the uniqueness of each case. Despite the uniqueness, however, the principles of treatment are consistent throughout, as is generally the outcome. The following story was first published in the *Heilkunst Journal*, and has been adapted for the book.

Gary's Story

Gary was diagnosed with autism at 22 months, and his parents watched for over six months as their son went from a happy, healthy child to a state of withdrawal from the world. The trigger? According to his mother, "Gary's decline coincided with a rash of ear infections and treatment with antibiotics, and followed vaccination with MMR and HI(b)."

Like most parents of autistic children, Gary's parents embarked on a long, tiring and mostly frustrating effort to find a way to bring their son back. Initially, they sought a solution within the conventional model, being trained in the sciences. They tried anything that had so-called rigorous double-blind randomized clinical trials.

The first step was to identify any chemical imbalances. He was found to be intolerant to wheat and dairy, and products containing phenols (food colorings, flavorings and preservatives). There was more.

> We discovered that of the four immunoglobulin G subclasses, he was deficient in two. We learned that certain fungal metabolites were so elevated in his blood, that he was surely fighting a huge systemic yeast overgrowth. We tested him for his body burden of toxins and found that he was laden with toxins – copper and zinc were elevated in his hair, and his chemical burden was very high.

Gary underwent a gamut of therapies – a restricted diet, bimonthly EPD (Enzyme Potentiated Desensitization) shots which required an even *more* restricted diet, intravenous IgG for three hours every month for fourteen months, antifungals for the yeast with a liver test every two months to monitor side-effects, visual therapy with prism lenses, Auditory Integration Therapy and Fast Forward Computer Therapy.

> For a period of three and a half years, we battled every symptom which could be identified by the medical community as somehow linked to Gary's problem.

But then deception settled in as the mother began to realize that her son was not really improving even though he had become a "poster child" for the American Society of Autism in terms of the drug treatments that were being tried. When asked to speak to the ASA's National Autism Convention, the mother felt that she could not in all honesty advocate to others the drug treatments her son was on, given the stark lack of results.

> Gary was completely disconnected from the world at this point, and my husband and I were gripped with fear. His behavior repertoire included a perseverative bouncing in his crib for as long as three hours at a stretch (if we let him), teeth grinding, guttural groaning sounds, and finger flapping in front of his eyes. Meanwhile he performed no eye contact, no appropriate toy play, no attachment behavior, and no pre-verbal gesturing like pointing.

Still, at this stage, they were only looking at "proven" therapies and opted for a three-year program of Dr. Ivar Lovaas's intensive discrete-trial behavior modification for up to thirty hours a week. Despite their hopes and hard work, Gary did not progress and, for the first time, his mother entertained the idea of stepping outside the conventional field to help her son.

The first step was detoxification using energized (so-called homeopathic) medicines in combinations. The results were initially good with reduced food sensitivities, elimination of the yeast overgrowth and increased awareness, but continued treatment after a year produced few additional gains compared with the periods of destabilization (healing reactions).

Next were visits to an osteopath to help release stress caused by the years of treatment and interventions. Again, healing reactions occurred (diarrhea, hyperactivity, and skin reactions) similar to those on the detox program.

Then the mother contacted our clinic on the recommendation of another parent. Given the earlier treatments, we started Gary on the sequential removal of diseases in the form of traumas during his life – from drugs and vaccinations to dental treatments and emotional stresses. The initial healing reactions were strong and often temporarily destabilizing, witness to the intensity of the shocks themselves to Gary's system. However, the results were rewarding.

> Six months after we started treatment, the veteran principal at the school that Gary attends approached me and told me that she had never seen such a dramatic change in a kid as she had witnessed in the past couple of months with Gary.

The pattern that emerged was one of a healing reaction followed by an overall increase in health as each trauma was removed. The traumas were removed, as is the case in sequential treatment, in the reverse order of their occurrence. By the time he arrived at the point of his birth in the timeline, Gary had been able to attend regular class, albeit with the help of an aide.

The next step in sequential treatment of disease is the removal of inherited weaknesses that are termed chronic miasms. These chronic miasms are like disease archetypes that give rise to all manner of symptoms and distortions of health, all of which conventional medicine gives an arbitrary name, ignorant of their common origin (see Annex A).

While it is not possible to use energetic medicines to alter the genetic code per se, it *is* possible to correct distortions in the functioning of the genes in terms of their folding and unfolding, which takes place in a fluid environment. The treatment is essentially the same for each person in terms of the medicines used and the sequence, but the reactions of each patient will vary according to the nature and degree of inherited weaknesses.

Since miasmic treatment starts to get at the root cause of most autistic cases, the healing reactions can be quite profound, as the body works to restore balance after the removal of a deep inherited blockage. Gary's case was no exception. At the end of the first round of miasmic treatment, however, significant changes occurred.

> He became much more aware of the people around him. He began to answer the telephone for the first time. One of the most profound memories for me from that time, less than a year ago, was while driving home from a meeting… I had left Gary at the house to play on his computer. I decided to call the house on the way home to check my messages.
>
> As the phone rang and I waited for my service to pick up, I was surprised by someone answering the phone with a shy, "Hello?" It was so off the map that Gary would answer the phone that I truly hadn't a clue who it was.
>
> "Who is this?" I asked.
>
> "It's Gary," he said quietly.
>
> I was so stunned that I couldn't really process what was going on.

"Hi, Gary. What are you doing?" I managed to whisper.

"I'm playing on the computer," he said.

"Are you okay?"

"Yes," he said.

"I'll see you soon, okay?"

"Okay. Bye Mommy."

It was such a leap, so much at once, that I couldn't really handle it. I managed to get my car to the side of the road through my tears and gave myself some time to absorb what had just happened.

Given the depth of Gary's condition, it was necessary to do several more rounds of treatment of the chronic miasms, each time at a higher level of energy (or potency, as we term it), which penetrated more deeply each time, removing deeper blockages. However, given the severity of his reaction to the first level, we decided to repeat the first level before starting on a second round. After the repeat of the first level, Gary was making substantial progress.

As the summer progressed, Gary became more and more stable. By the time school started, I had a strong sense that we were left only with a game of catch-up. He was far behind his same-aged peers in social skills, but he was closing the gap steadily… I was blown away by his new cognitive ability. It was as if, over the summer, new neurological pathways had developed. He was able to master skills that were unapproachable at the end of the previous academic year.

…Now suddenly I was sitting with a boy who could simply understand what I was saying. It was a huge leap that had occurred over the course of a summer during which he had no formal schooling.

…I had a strong sense that we were in a game of catch-up now and that there was an element of autopilot to the whole thing. Where before I felt pivotal to the process –

> that without my constant monitoring, pushing and adjusting he would not make it – I started to get the feeling that he would be okay now, regardless of my intervention.

Next it was time to go into the second round of the chronic miasms, or inherited diseases. Each of the rounds acts at a specific level of the human organism, going progressively deeper into the interior and closer to the true roots of the problem. The depth of the roots of the autistic condition in any given case will vary and is not known in advance. However, it is fair to say that the roots of disease behind each autistic condition are quite deep and extensive.

That is why there is limited improvement from many therapies in most cases, as these therapies can only correct imbalances (using the law of opposites), but cannot remove disease. It is *only* when you systematically attack the diseases lying behind the autistic condition on the basis of the law of similars, while simultaneously supporting the patient with various therapies to help re-balance feelings, functions and sensations that you can expect, and will receive, significant improvement.

In Gary's case going deeper was essential. He had improved, but was not out of the woods yet by any means. The second round brought up a strong healing reaction, and also opened the door to a new realm of disease that we call the "chthonic realm."

Chthonic is the Greek word for "earth." This is the realm of fear and anxiety. Behavior driven by fear is highly irrational and destructive. In the case of children, we see a range of behavior that is wild, defiant, scatological, self-destructive, violent, threatening and delusional. It can also involve somewhat the opposite: pathological shyness, need to control, obsessive-compulsive behavior, and a complete lack of awareness of self and one's surroundings. In this range of behaviors, we can see the roots of many of the behavioral conditions of children these days, which are given arbitrary labels such as ADD, ADHD, ODD, PDD, autism, etc., labels that describe, but do not provide any insights into effective treatment.

In Heilkunst, thanks to our own research and clinical experience using the principles of natural law, we have been able to map the chthonic realm and identify effective remedies for each of the sub-states within this realm. It is a realm of fear, pure and simple. All of the behavior that we witness coming from this realm is driven by an intense fear, a fear of losing control over one's inner sensations, of being swept along in a powerful current and losing touch with reality.

The essential problem with autistic children is that they have a tenuous grip on external reality (lack of awareness) and are too closely connected to the natural, irrational realm within themselves. They do not have the filter most of us have, thanks to our human evolution over the centuries, to separate themselves from nature. In a very real sense autistic children are living in an earlier state of human consciousness, one that had us living intimately with and in nature, with little distinction of self (self-consciousness).

At one level, this provides for a high degree of creativity because they are directly in touch with the well-springs of genius, with little censoring of this natural source by their intellect or rational mind. On the other hand, it means that they have difficulty connecting with the rest of us, since we live for the most part in a profound separation from our deeper, inner self. We have a strong sense of self that is the product of this separation from nature. We are still subject to irrational behavior, we still have hunches, gut feelings, inspirations and intuitions, but this is not the norm as it was thousands of years ago.

In an evolutionary sense we have crossed over a divide that provides an almost unbridgeable chasm between us and nature. For some reason autistic children have gone back over to the other side, and we have lost contact with them, and they with us.

This state of living in an earlier, more primitive state of consciousness is often hidden in terms of its overt expression. All that is seen is the general expression of this state in terms of the "escape from reality." Then it is given a descriptive label, often from Greek or Latin (and in this case, the term "autism"), a label that hides more than it reveals.

However, as treatment approaches the lair of the beast, so to speak, fear comes out in all its various forms. It is simply a more definitive expression of something that has been there all along, as parents come to realize.

> ...I have a strong sense that [the chthonic realm] is as big a part of Gary's autism as the miasms were/are... I realized that it was a state Gary had flirted with constantly for the past eight years. I also realized that when we effectively banish it for good, Gary will emerge a much freed individual.

8| The Meaning of Autism

The Separation of Self

Seeing the roots of autism in the realm of primordial fear leads us to the beginnings of an understanding of autism and why it is emerging in such numbers in our time. We can either take life's happenings as the "chance whirlings of random particles," or accept that there is pattern and meaning in all of life. If there is meaning in just *one* part of life, and we can all attest to that, then we must accept that there is meaning in *all* of Creation, even if we do not know what that might be in a given case.

In an evolutionary sense we have gradually separated from nature, from what the Bible calls the tree of life. As a result of the emergence of the intellect, which gave us a sense of our self, we have a separation from the primordial state of being. This is given to us in the form of the tasting of fruit from the tree of knowledge. The world of instinctual, primordial nature, the tree of life, we are not given to know; it remains hidden from our view behind veils created by our sense of self, our self-consciousness, what the Bible calls the "fading splendor."

We can see the result of this epic development in human evolution everywhere around us. We live in a world created almost entirely out of the mind of man, driven by technology and the rules of the intellect (linear logic and linear time), a world that has effectively lost touch with its inner self, the world of instinct, intuition, imagination and inspiration.

Only the very few, thc geniuses among us in both science and art, are able to make the perilous passage back to the other shore and then return alive to report on the wonders and treasures lying there to the rest of us who are not adventuresome enough or do not have the discipline, training or courage to go to the edge of the known world ourselves. We depend on our artists to keep the wellsprings of creativity from drying up and our culture from dying of a new form of arteriosclerosis, like hardening of the attitudes.

Much of the official society that we live in, dominated by a material form of science, has rejected the world on the other shore as either non-existent or off-limits (occult, meaning beyond). Our outer lives are ruled by our intellect (our brain mind), but our inner lives, at the personal level, are unconsciously driven by our gut, or body mind. To a very real degree we all live between our conscious mind and actions and our unconscious needs and desires, between Apollo and Dionysius. Art fulfills our needs to some extent, but we are also driven to irrational behavior to keep some balance.

Ancient societies understood better that there needed to be a regular outlet for our instinctual self, and this was reflected in various times when restraint and reason were allowed to be overrun by instinctual desires in the form of events such as revelries, carnivals and bacchanalias. Our society faces the same need for instinctual expression, but our instinctual, natural self is continually at war with our conscious, rational self. The two are not acting in harmony.

The solution is not a continual tug-of-war, or ever-wider swinging of the pendulum from rational, consciously-controlled to wild, unconsciously-controlled behavior, but a more integrated state of the two aspects of our being. This requires nothing less than that we bring the hitherto hidden and often denied world of the supersensible (that is, the world beyond the senses) back into our conscious life (into our science) and into harmony with the way that we live. If not we'll continue to live a dual life, a form of cultural schizophrenia. As the rational side of us grows in strength, the so-called irrational side must become even stronger to maintain balance.

9| Our Evolution of Consciousness

In an evolutionary sense, we are moving from one stage of human consciousness to another. We are currently in the process of converting our inner world of feeling and desire (what in the esoteric literature is called the astral body, as it involves the stars – de-sire meaning "from the stars") – into a more spiritual form. This means that our astral body, our inner world of feeling, is more vulnerable to outside influences.

In order to change we have to open ourselves to the possibility of change. Over the past several decades, we have become more sensitive in terms of our feelings, but this has also been reflected at the level of our functions and sensations (our energetic and physical levels respectively).

From this we have a whole phenomenon of hyperactivity – from allergic reactions and environmental sensitivities to an inability to focus and concentrate (ADD, ADHD). During this phase of change we become more vulnerable to various shocks and traumas, like vaccinations, chemicals, drugs and the process of change itself (moves, family disruptions, career changes, technological advances). Our children are born with a greater propensity *for* change, but also with a greater capacity to be affected *by* change and outside events.

As a society we are reaching out from the conscious world of our rational mind, which increasingly dominates, to try to find balance in the supersensible world, that world which is beyond our senses. However, too often this search is not done in harmony with our conscious self, but almost in opposition to it.

What we have then is the creation of a polarity between the product of our rational mind, as material "science" (that studies only the appearances of nature or *natura naturata*) and the product of our instinctual mind as mystical "science" (that seeks to find the hidden essence of nature or *natura naturans*).

This polarity only divides, it does not integrate. We simply have two solitudes, where "never the 'twain shall meet." The solution is *not* to go in the opposite direction from the materialist, rational direction of our modern culture, and into the escape of mysticism. We need to struggle to *understand* the supersensible world (the world beyond our sense experience), the one that lies within us and is used in our personal life, but is not recognized as legitimate in our public and professional life.

This struggle must involve our conscious, rational mind, so that we remain fully aware of what we are exploring, thereby making it a true science. However, to do so we must remove the cultural and evolutionary split within ourselves, the one between our two minds and selves – our rational, brain mind living in our conscious self (the tree of knowledge), and our instinctual, body mind, living in our unconscious self (the tree of life).

To do so requires that we be healthy, as disease blocks any integration of our two sides and prevents us from becoming free spirits. To be fully integrated (healthy) is to be free from the prison of fear and illusion. Fear is the product of our instinctual self, living in an unrefined state of nature, separated from our rational self.

Illusion and delusion are the products of our rational self, living in the sensible world and separated from our inner knowing (wisdom). We can only know the *appearance* of things in Western philosophy and science, not the thing itself.

10| The New Plague

Autism in children has become like a plague upon the land. Epidemic disturbances reflect the particular state of society in time and the spiritual struggles that mankind is going through. It seems that the emerging generation of autistic children are themselves confronting, and forcing adults to confront, the need to find integration between our rational self and our oft-ignored and denigrated, if not outright denied, instinctual self, the realm of our wisdom. We have become, over the centuries, estranged from this wisdom, and our over-developed and dominating rational, conscious self cannot truly know anything beyond the material world of the senses.

The state of our own self, with its profound inner split, is mirrored for us in our children. Like the canary in the coal mine, the so-called autistic children are warning us of the dangers of the path we are on as a society and the need to struggle to find the path to the integration, in full consciousness, of both worlds within us. We cannot escape into denial, living purely in the material world; nor can we escape into mysticism, seeking to live purely in the super-sensible world. We must live in both, harmoniously.

Gary's mother became fully aware of this during Gary's treatment. She realized that *she* also needed to be treated, and that her son's release from his autistic state would be hampered so long as she lived in a state of being split from her self.

Both parents were trained in material science and first sought out that which could be explained on its terms, but his mother then came increasingly to understand the need to trust her inner wisdom and to see that the struggle with autism was a profound conscious journey into trust and love. As her son became more whole, so did she, and as she became more integrated within herself, so too did her son find his way back into the sensible world.

We intended to fight this thing [autism] and win... I approached this research with an eye to science. Interventions which had been subjected to rigorous "scientific" study, and had gained approval through the process of peer-review, were more palatable to both my husband and me. Our upbringing and education had, I thought, well prepared us for this obstacle. At this point in our crusade, our intuition was not even a close second to the influence of the "scientific community."

...My rainbow-chasing days were drawing to a close, however, as I began to realize that in spite of our frantic efforts, my intuition was telling me that Gary was not really improving...

Three years into our crusade, cracks were appearing in the wall which we had so fearfully erected between the world of "science" and the world beyond. If we were to make any sustained, sure progress with Gary, it was clear we would have to leave the world of fear behind us and venture into the world of faith [trust]...

Meanwhile, my approach to Gary at home began to change... I no longer put much stock in the "experts" on my son's condition as I began to support him in the direction of his own natural development...

As my own fear began to slip away, I learned to relax my need for control, and I have put Gary's future in his own hands, where it belongs...

As I thrashed around trying to find some light, I realized that I was facing another big lesson. I was clearly far too attached to the outcome, to Gary's recovery... It was as if the universe was telling me that surely Gary couldn't be done yet, because I still had a ways to go myself...

I find that the healthier I grow, the less inclined I am to share Gary's progress in terms of the way the diseased world thinks – autism vs. normal, or recovered. It is far more complicated than that, and the lessons we are learning along the way are more profound.

11| Heilkunst and the Gift of Autism

Autism in a child is a deep shock and struggle for the parent, and yet it is hard to escape the conclusion that it is a gift of love from the universe. We are offered a compelling opportunity to venture on a profound and necessary journey to the heart of darkness within our soul in order to rescue the child lost beyond the veil of our sense-limited world. This journey takes courage and trust and forces us to confront our own limitations, both as parent and practitioner.

The good news is that the medical science of Heilkunst offers a means of undertaking the journey into the darkness to confront our fears and illusions, and ensures we will return safe and sound, albeit profoundly changed in our relationship to our self and the world around us. The means are founded on and derived from natural law and only serve to remove unnecessary blockages to the journey we must undertake.

While each case is unique, being the journey of unique individuals, the principles are universal and can be applied to any case. The outcome is, in equal parts, both unique and universal. If we act according to natural law then the outcome is consistently positive.

The degree of integration of any child into the sense world that we now largely inhabit will, of course, vary depending on numerous factors, some of which for now lie beyond the capacity to encompass them in our current state of human evolution. For now each child and each case provides us with the opportunity to extend the frontier of our knowing, a true integration of our rational mind with our inner wisdom (body mind), and with it our ability to help those, both adults and children, struggling with their individual integration of self.

12| Case Studies

The snippets and cases interspersed throughout the pages of this book, as well as those shown below, represent a number of our current cases. They are intended to illustrate the diversity of situations, as well as the common factors, in autistic conditions. The cases are all at different stages in treatment and all have shown varied amounts of treatment time before improvement was evident.

But what they share is that they have *all* seen significant benefits during treatment with Heilkunst. Of course, results cannot be attributed solely to our work, as in some cases various therapies were used prior to and during these cases. Our hope and continued wish is for a more integrated and comprehensive plan for the treatment of autism. We feel strongly that Heilkunst offers this possibility in a way that nothing else ever has, or ever can.

Brad's Story

Brad's case, as set out in considerable detail, is useful as it shows clearly the benefits at a deep level of the sequential clearance of various shocks and traumas, particularly from vaccinations. Often parents are trying many other therapies with their child during sequential treatment, and are not sure what is causing improvements. In a sense, all approaches help to some degree, but it is our experience and assessment at the Hahnemann Clinic for Heilkunst that the use of homeopathic medicines to clear various shocks provides a degree of cure of underlying causes of autism that is *not possible* using any other approach, particularly in severe and resistant cases.

This case also clearly demonstrates the logic and natural law basis for a sequential approach, as that is the direction the body's own natural healing force wishes to follow. By respecting the body's own cues and direction, Heilkunst homeopathic treatment is *much* more effective, compared to trying to impose a treatment based on a rather arbitrary decision as to what to treat and when.

As is the case here, Brad had been treated for various vaccination shocks, but with little improvement. This illustrates the maxim of the sequential order of treatment: It is not enough to have the right remedy, you must give the right remedy in the right potency at the right time.

At the Hahnemann Clinic for Heilkunst, we also feel strongly that the traumas to the child should be minimized, and that travel and dislocation from the usual surroundings and routines can add to trauma. We also feel that treatment should be accessible to all, and Heilkunst treatment can largely be done over the phone, without having seen the child, relying on the timeline of shocks and information about the child from the parent(s). This also considerably reduces the cost of treatment to the parents, while not reducing in any way the benefits to the child.

The deep fear and sexually suggestive nature of the underlying world behind the autistic condition that renders some children so easily destabilized is here brought out very clearly. In a sense, vaccinations delivered in the conventional way, in crude form, simply act as a trigger, all the more with these children due to their high sensitivity to heavy metals, in particular thimerosal/mercury.

However, we also have seen cases of deep aggression, sexual lewdness and general out-of-control behavior in children who had never been vaccinated, which supports that the vaccinations bring *out* the problem, but that the problem lies deeper in the inherited realm. What will benefit autistic children will also benefit other children with behavioral problems.

The strong nature of the healing reactions in physical terms, such as the diarrhea and the recurrent facial rash, is not typical, but does illustrate the need for the body to discharge the toxins produced by shocks to the system, resulting at the same time in overall improvement in the mental/emotional state of the child. We have not commented in more detail on the treatment in this case, as the parental comments have essentially captured the process.

Parent's Assessment

We have been treating our son, Brad, through the Hahnemann Clinic for Heilkunst for about 18 months at the time of writing this report. In this period, he has completed the treatment of the various shocks and traumas on his timeline and has gone through one full round of the chronic miasms, or inherited disease tendencies. He is just beginning his second round of miasms. In this time, he has experienced many ups and downs, but overall, more "ups" than with any other treatments we have tried previously, and we have tried many things.

Brad is nine years old, which is considered "old" by the standards of practitioners who treat autism – both mainstream and alternative. To give you some of the background, Brad was diagnosed with autism at the age of two and a half. Until he was almost five, we stuck with the mainstream therapies available, which included ABA (Applied Behavior Analysis), which is an intensive form of behavioral teaching, Speech Therapy, and Occupational Therapy with a Sensory Integration component.

To start with, let me tell you what he was like as a young child. Brad exhibited extreme mechanical brilliance as a young toddler. By the age of 19 months, his favorite pastime was dismantling his entire crib by taking the bolts apart with his bare fingers. (For those in the know, one of the characteristics of autism in young children is the lack of ordinary play skills. Children with autism tend to play with toys inappropriately or find other strange things to do to pass the time.) We just thought he was a genius, and had no inkling that this was a sign of autism. So adept was he in the mechanical domain, that at the age of two and a half, at his first appointment with the Chief of Developmental Pediatrics at our Children's Hospital, he fascinated the doctor by figuring out how to pick the lock on her office door and escaping down the hall.

He was extremely hyperactive, would always bolt and run away if not restrained, and had no concept of danger. He would turn on the stove and then climb up and sit on it; he would run into traffic if not restrained. He would pick his nose and gums until they bled. He would bite his wrists whenever he was anxious, and so they were black and blue from his cutting the skin with his teeth. He had extreme sound sensitivities and would cover his ears and lie down on the ground screaming at the sound of the food processor, vacuum cleaner, or coffee grinder.

He needed to be supervised 24/7. His behavior problems were so severe that the psychologist we brought up from California recommended staffing our home-based ABA program with aides four or five evenings per week in addition to daytime shifts, just to help us cope with and train us in how to teach our son adaptive living skills.

At the age of three, he used to smear his feces every night in his bedroom and grind them into the carpet, dump all his clothes out of his drawers, smear it all over his clothes, his bed, the walls, and later himself. Mealtime was just as challenging. He would shove food into his mouth with his hands, dump it all over the floor, spill everyone's water, and run around the table and try to choke me from behind.

The fun continued at bath time where he would splash tons of water onto the floor, chew everyone's toothbrush he could get his hands on (we had to lock up all our toothbrushes!), and often squeeze out entire tubes of toothpaste and other bathroom products onto the carpet.

So, we definitely needed some help to manage all of this, and had a team of as many as seven therapists/aides at a time in our home back in those days. I am not even sure how many aides have worked in our home program over the last seven years; I lost count after 40. This very necessary help also added to the lack of privacy our family had and to all of the problems of being an employer in one's own home. And you can imagine what all of this can do to a family's social life, marriage, and sibling relationships.

Every child is an individual, and that goes for every child with autism as well. The stereotypical view of classic autism includes a child who rocks back and forth, is antisocial, is unaffectionate and doesn't like to be held. None of this could ever have been used to describe Brad. He was always social, just inappropriately so. He always had some language; he just didn't use it meaningfully. And he was always affectionate towards his family.

At the same time, as a young child, his behavior was extremely challenging. By the age of four, he had broken all the furniture in our living room, with the exception of our piano and two couches. Almost every day between 4:00 and 6:00 p.m., he would have a massive temper tantrum where, in a matter of seconds, he would escalate from being a sweet little boy to a wild animal. He would go into a complete meltdown on the floor, kicking, hitting, biting, scratching, throwing objects, knocking things down, and slamming doors so hard that all our walls had holes in them from the door handles.

In addition to all of the above, he developed many irrational fears – of vacuum cleaners, and especially of bedroom slippers that had faces or depicted animals or cartoon characters – all of which terrified him. He also developed strong obsessive-compulsive tendencies and many ritualistic behaviors, such as having to watch the credits in their entirety at the end of videos. If any of these and other rituals were interrupted or disturbed, it would always lead to a massive temper tantrum of the sort described above.

Near the end of 1999, I was surfing the Net on autism sites, and came across one on the GFCF (gluten-free, casein-free) diet for autism. When I scrolled down the site to read about the markers to look for to know if your child was a candidate for this diet, Brad had nine out of 10 of them!

We next embarked on the world of special diets. The first thing I did was remove dairy and all packaged processed foods that contained any form of casein or whey powder as an ingredient. Within 24 hours, the melt down tantrums, which lasted at least an hour and were almost daily, decreased in frequency to about once every two weeks, and even then, with the edge removed. He started falling asleep more quickly at night. It became easier to reason with him, and numerous other improvements, all from just removing dairy!

We later experimented with removing all gluten, then a yeast-free diet in addition, the Feingold diet, and much later still, the Specific Carbohydrate Diet which is a grain-free, starch-free, and yeast-free diet. All of these diets helped him in different ways.

Through other parents on Internet chat groups and through word-of-mouth, I learned of and tried many other treatments, including a barrage of medical tests that included shipping Brad's urine, saliva, blood, and feces to various labs in the U.S., Auditory Integration Therapy, Fast For Word computer programming to assist with expressive and receptive language, EEG Biofeedback, nutritional supplements, antifungals and other aspects of the DAN! Protocol (Defeat Autism Now! Protocol developed by MDs who are interested in trying new treatments that haven't necessarily passed 20-year clinical trials), detoxification, Reiki, cranio-sacral therapy, NAET, and several kinds of homeopathy.

By the time I found out about the sequential approach to using homeopathic medicines and the Hahnemann Clinic, I was already a battle-weary veteran on the long journey in search of a "cure" for my son. Why did I choose this treatment over others? There were a number of reasons.

For one thing, we had exhausted our life savings, undertaken expensive travel and long distance treatments with various practitioners in different parts of the U.S. We had had remedies lost in the mail, held up at Canada Customs, and incurred extensive waiting periods to receive treatments, not to mention costly shipping and custom duties. So, to find a practitioner with a special interest and expertise in treating autism here in Canada, where we live, was very compelling, as well as the possibility to do much if not all of the consultations over the phone and via the internet.

Many parents undertake this use of homeopathic medicine in conjunction with mercury chelation and various other types of alternative medical treatments with the feeling that homeopathy is not sufficient, or because they are hedging their bets that the more treatments they throw at their child at once, the better the chances that something will work eventually.

While it is easy to understand the desperation that parents feel, for me, personally, after so many years of so many intensive therapies, and so many thousands of dollars and thousands of hours of time and energy expended, it made sense to now follow one main approach. While I continue to give my son a handful of nutritional supplements, and carry on with cranio-sacral therapy which I believe complements his sequential treatment by helping the healing take place, I have ceased trying every new "flavor of the month."

The other more important reasons why we are staying the course with this treatment are that it goes much deeper than any other treatment I am aware of or have experienced. What I mean is that it not only addresses the toxins, gastrointestinal problems and other physical symptoms associated with autism, it also addresses emotional and spiritual issues, and digs down to the core or essence of each patient. For my own child, I see this reflected in the fact that the remedies for various traumas seem to trigger deep healing reactions. Many of these reactions appear to be coming from the subconscious or from some very deep primordial place within him. While it is not an easy journey, the improvements we see after each of these healing crises give us the impression that he is healing from the inside out.

The first trauma on Brad's timeline was for the chicken pox virus that he had contracted a couple years ago. Together with the NSOL and constitutional remedy, *Sulphur*, there was also a homeopathic remedy for anxiety in his initial dropper bottle. Within a week or two, we saw significant improvements in his behavior that could only be attributed to his sequential treatment.

He seemed more attentive at school, better able to concentrate, and even began putting up his hand when his grade two teacher asked questions, and responding with appropriate, correct answers when called upon. This had never occurred before on his own initiative without prompting from his aide. His extreme anxiety, especially after school and in the early evening, was much reduced. And best of all, the aggression faded to almost nothing, and this from a boy who used to hit or kick me (and others) 20 times a day on average. There were so many immediate marked improvements that when I had my first follow-up phone consultation a month later, my Heilkünstler was very surprised and felt certain that these remedies must have removed a blockage that allowed the potential benefits of all the other treatments we had been doing for years manifest more effectively and fully.

The remedy for chicken pox was followed by one for the negative (so-called side) effects of Diflucan, the antifungal we had tried through an alternative MD, then remedies for an accident where Brad had fallen off the top of our china cabinet (he was a climber) and pierced his scrotum on the edge of the stereo speaker, and next a remedy for a bad flu with a high fever that had lasted several days. What was so interesting to me was the fact that he would start going through reactions to the next trauma often a week or so before actually taking the remedy to remove that trauma. So, for example, he got flu-like symptoms including lethargy and fever several days before we administered the remedy for the flu. While in all the above-mentioned cases, there were some mild reactions, they seemed to cycle through him quickly and continued to bring on-going further improvements.

So, by the end of the summer of 2003, five months into treatment, we had seen considerable progress. We actually had been able to go out as a family to two crowded barbeque events with no aide along to assist us. We considered both events a huge success because he didn't hit, kick, or spit at anyone, he didn't attempt to run away, and he didn't sneak any forbidden foods. We hadn't ever been able to pull anything like this off, and considered it the first successful family endeavor in six years!

I was now able to take Brad shopping to the supermarket without much incident. Prior to starting sequential treatment, if we would run into anyone Brad knew at the supermarket, the library, or the mall, he would get extremely upset because his rigid mind told him they weren't supposed to be there. He would either scream when they said hello to him, or he would run away, or hit them or me. Suddenly, he was able to greet people he knew at the supermarket or store quietly and appropriately.

Talking on the phone for me was always a huge challenge because Brad would shout continually that he wanted to talk to the person. If I would actually give him the phone, he would either shout inappropriate comments into the receiver, or he would run away. But he would never allow me to carry on a conversation. This problem was now alleviated.

In addition, we noticed that some of his fears, rigidities, and OCD tendencies had been reduced. For instance, for years he always insisted that his cupboard drawer door remain open, as he was afraid of what might lurk behind it if it were closed. All of a sudden, he was tolerating having it closed. He seemed less fearful of slippers, and would sometimes even tolerate passing them in the aisles of department stores without screaming.

However, this rather mild ebb and flow of reactions to his trauma remedies followed by continued improvements changed dramatically a year ago August when we hit the vaccine traumas on his timeline. I had anticipated severe reactions at the DTaP (Diptheria, Tetanus, Pertussis),

Polio, and MMR (Measles, Mumps, Rubella) booster shots that Brad had received at age four and a half because his regression at the time of the vaccines was severe.

While he had reactions, they were not all that strong. My practitioner told me after the fact that the very high potencies had not been used with these ones because they were mainly boosters, not the original vaccination shock. Nonetheless, some of his old behavioral problems resurfaced. These included flushing bars of soap down the toilet, aggression, and spitting at people. These were all behaviors he had actively been engaged in at the age of the actual vaccine booster shots, surely no coincidence.

He also developed a distinct raw, red rash on his face, wakefulness until midnight, and intense perseverative talking about his past transgressions. At the same time, his sense of humor seemed to be developing more.

The next trauma remedy was for the vaccines he had had at the age of 18 months, which included DPT, polio, and HI(b) Influenza. At 18 months of age, the day he received these vaccines, I can remember attending a barbeque that evening. Brad was in his stroller. I undid the straps to let him out. I suppose the shifting and movement triggered pain from the shot. His crying and screaming lasted over an hour. At the time I realized he was crying from the pain of the needle, but I had no idea that he was suffering a "vaccine adverse reaction."

So, it was no surprise that he had a strong healing reaction following the homeopathic remedy, but we were unprepared for the extent of its severity. At first his father took the brunt of it. One day, about a week after ingesting the remedy, and after being told not to stand so close to the T.V., Brad began hitting his father in the head as forcefully as he could, shouting and screaming.

His behavior worsened at school, and for the next two weeks he was spitting at, poking, and shoving his classmates, and was loud, hyper, and inattentive. This culminated in a day when he had a meltdown tantrum and stripped his shirt off, and lay down on the floor in the middle of his classroom while his teacher was instructing.

Around the same time, during car rides with me, he began undoing his seatbelt, flailing around the back seat, and hitting and kicking me while I was driving – a common occurrence when he was three or four years old. (This behavior problem had been eliminated at that age through intensive behavioral intervention.) At the same time, he developed that same deep, red, raw rash on his cheeks, nose, and chin, and the same rash could be found on his thumb which he began sucking. He also developed chronic, foul-smelling, explosive diarrhea, of the consistency of brown water. This diarrhea continued unabated for six months.

One day he went for his monthly appointment with his cranio-sacral therapist. When I came to pick him up, the therapist related that during the treatment, Brad had begun crying like a baby, and shouting that the needle was hurting him. The therapist had not been informed that Brad was detoxing his 18-month vaccines.

This incident amazed me, and proved not only how powerful sequential homeopathic treatment is, but how profoundly it works, on the subconscious and other deep, emotional levels. We had detoxed Brad for his vaccines three times before, in three different kinds of treatments with three different homeopaths. We had seen immense healing reactions each time, but nothing of this deeper, subconscious level reaction and clearing.

With the next trauma remedy, the MMR vaccine, given at one year old, we saw many reactions as well, although not as severe as with the 18-month vaccine remedies. This surprised me because in retrospect (although I was completely unaware of it at the time), Brad began his descent into autism about three months after receiving the MMR vaccine. A seemingly healthy, normally developing infant at about 15 months of age, he stopped responding to his name when called. I can remember at 16 months carrying him upright to place him in his car seat. I recall holding him and saying, "I love you, Brad." He responded, "I love you too, Mommy." I never heard those words again for the next two years. After that incident, his behavior became increasingly hyperactive, and odd. I now believe that the 18-month vaccines intensified his downward spiral, worsening his condition.

The pocket of trauma we hit continued on with the MMR remedy, and extended on downward. Immediately after taking this remedy, Brad developed a cold and cough that lasted three weeks. This cough was also a detoxing discharge, and a form of healing reaction. A few days after taking the remedy, he started having some very challenging behavior during parts of each day.

What was interesting, though, was that after hitting or kicking me or his therapist, he would show remorse afterwards and begin crying because he felt ashamed and guilty for hurting us. We had never observed this kind of remorse in him before. Once again, the raw, red rash broke out all over his cheeks, nose, and chin. The rash was so severe this time that his aide at school told me the teachers were asking if he was allergic to something. I responded to her by saying yes, he was allergic to vaccines!

There were several days both at school and at home where he would curl up in the fetal position on the floor, and sometimes strip off his clothes from the waist up. After 15 minutes or so on the floor, this would always be followed by an incident of aggression and other odd behavior. It almost seemed as though he was trying to get back into the womb, or in touch with his pre-birth self. At the same time, he became very verbally abusive, and would tell his aide that he wanted "to puke" on her, and tell his father that he wanted to rip off his glasses, and other things of that nature.

Off and on throughout the treatment, his extreme sensitivity to sounds has returned, even to the point where he often cannot tolerate the sound of the toilet flushing. His gums have been bleeding off and on as well, another detoxing discharge reaction. Between these various incidents, however, he has seen further improvements in both his behavior and academic skills. At his monthly craniosacral therapy appointment, his therapist said his liver and kidneys were hot and that there was a lot of buzzing and movement in the left side of his brain. At the same appointment, he built a large, complex Lego structure. This is the first time in his life that he constructed something out of Lego by himself that was anything other than a flat square.

About two weeks after taking the MMR remedy, Brad exposed himself at recess to three girls from his school. This kind of thing had never happened before. When the school principal called, she said that if it had been any other boy, he would have automatically been suspended, but because it was Brad, with his disability, that would not be the case, but they wanted him to leave for that afternoon.

When I called the Hahnemann Clinic office, they made some adjustments to Brad's remedies, yet this incident was followed by two similar incidents when we had company at our home. My practitioner said this sexually-oriented behavior was likely coming from somewhere very deep within Brad, a realm of deep fear common to autistic children, which is known in Heilkunst as the chthonic realm. Completely mortified, several months later when I met another practitioner who specializes in autism at the Hahnemann Clinic and recounted this event, the comment that I should be happy he was going through this now instead of at the age of 20 gave me a new perspective on the matter!

A week later I administered the trauma remedies for the two, four, and six-month vaccines combined. They were combined because they were all for DPT, Polio, and HI(b) Influenza, and there were no other traumas that occurred in between. He had a very good couple of days immediately after taking the remedies, but then the problems started a couple days later. He started telling classmates that he wanted to kill them, and that their penises had fallen off. He became much more hyperactive and unfocussed at school. There were further incidents at home of him curling up in the fetal position and aggressing. He became louder, more boisterous, and was often pushing and shoving kids at school.

For weeks on end, Brad began climbing into his sister's bed in the middle of the night and sleeping with her, stating that he was afraid to be alone in the dark. He began obsessing over his indecent exposure incidents, and while they have never reoccurred, he has been talking about them a great deal ever since. Around this time, his bowel movements, still watery, took on a golden hue. The rash that erupted on his face following these last vaccines was of a milder sort than on previous rounds. A few weeks after taking the remedies, he had a tummy ache and threw up during the night. He had no fever, and seemed fine in the morning.

Other sexual overtones started appearing. He seemed to have an inordinate interest in the grade 4 and 5 girls at his school who were a year or two older. He was constantly trying to hang around them and would ask them embarrassing questions about their breasts. One day after school when I was reading his aide's notes to me in his Communication notebook, I found out that he had gotten kicked out of gym class that day for going up to a girl and kissing her on the lips. When I asked him at bedtime why he had done this, he replied, "The needle went through me." When I tried to probe for more information, I got no further explanation – another enigmatic example of deep sexual feelings brought out by the vaccination shocks, which seem to trigger this deeper realm of fear that encompasses inappropriate sexual behavior.

He experienced several days with a lot of emotional outbursts, recollecting past misdemeanors, and grieving over old friends and classmates who had moved away or left his school. In the aftermath of his vaccine remedies, we did notice some marked gains in expressive language, a bit less inappropriate talking, and more on-topic conversation, with some improvements in grammar and syntax. The rashes on his face came and went several more times, and his skin was very dry and chapped. He was constantly opening his mouth very wide, as if his ears were blocked and he was making vain attempts to clear them.

His next trauma was a course of antibiotics he had had for an ear infection at four weeks old. We didn't see any major reactions to this one. After the second night of remedy powders for his circumcision, he began shouting and hitting me on the head and the next morning he scratched me repeatedly. He assaulted the janitor at his school when he held the door open for us. He began shouting at some of his classmates that he was going to cut off their penises. Talk about the subconscious rising to the surface!

That evening in the bath he started shouting and crying that he was going to slit so-and-so's throat and cut off their head. His language was very violent for a period of time, and it took some time for him to calm down again. The next evening he had about an hour and a half where he was hitting us, kicking, screaming, spitting in our faces, throwing objects – in short, completely out of control. Where his healing reactions usually occurred one to two weeks after taking a remedy, with the circumcision trauma remedy, the reactions were almost immediate, leading me to believe the destabilization the event had caused must have been very close to the surface.

The next morning it seemed to have disappeared completely from his system, and we were left with our sweet little boy again. When my husband asked him in the morning what had happened to him the night before, he responded in wide-eyed wonder, "I don't know," as if he was truly puzzled by his own behavior.

As my Heilkünstler had suggested might occur, Brad had an echo effect of this same reaction, of shorter and milder duration about a week later, lasting an hour or so several days in a row. When I had my next phone consult, my practitioner seemed rather surprised to hear of the strong reaction Brad had had to the circumcision remedies, explaining that most males get a slight rash for a few days and that this is the extent of their detoxing reaction. It was posited that autistic children are super-sensitive and react strongly and become particularly destabilized by events such as these that occur early in their lives, as is the case with the Hepatitis B vaccination given at birth or shortly thereafter in many states of the United States.

Brad must have felt under assault at the time of the event. This also made sense to me since at the time of the actual event, the person doing the circumcision sort of botched things up, Brad lost a lot of blood, and it took an inordinate amount of time to complete.

After this time, he experienced some improvements in asserting his independence. He had a classmate over for a play date. His aide had to leave early and the boys wanted to continue to play together. They did so quietly, in our basement with no adult intervention for four hours! I can remember phoning a friend and leaving her a voice mail message telling her that for the first time in six years I felt just like a typical mom of a typical child having a regular play date with a typical friend.

Next, he had two birth traumas to take. One was for the actual birth, and the other was for the amniocentesis and ultrasounds I had had during my pregnancy. Just as he would sometimes experience reactions to remedies before being given them, he would, at times, start having challenging behaviors that could be a sign that he was ready for the next remedy. This was the case when it was time to move on to the birth remedies.

He threw a scale down and broke it at school one day when he didn't like what his aide was telling him. He started biting himself and caused bruising again – something we hadn't seen in several years. So, I decided to give him the first birth remedy a week ahead of schedule as I suspected he was ready for it. Sure enough, there were immediate improvements by the next day. He was better focused, more compliant, and even his handwriting improved. He became much more appropriately affectionate to me, and very helpful around the house – folding laundry, loading the dishwasher.

A few days later, he had an all-day program with his Cubs pack at a museum. He behaved very well the entire day and even tolerated assistance from the volunteers there who helped him adjust a historic reproduction costume that he had tried on. This really amazed me because he has always been extremely rigid about letting anybody touch him or help him with anything like that, especially people he didn't know. As always, this was followed a few days later by the red rash on his face. Around the same time, his stool finally changed from stinky brown water to mashed potato consistency with the occasional formed stool.

The final trauma on his timeline was for mercury. When I was seven weeks pregnant I contracted a bad cold. Knowing I was pregnant, I went into a drugstore and asked the pharmacist what would be safe for me to take to relieve the congestion I was experiencing. He had recommended nasal drops in saline solution. Many years later, I learned that these saline drops usually contain thimerosal, the same mercury-based preservative found in many vaccines, that has been suspected of triggering autism, ADD, tics, and other learning disabilities.

Once again, the day after receiving the mercury remedy, we observed immediate improvements. Brad began handling disappointments better, such as dealing with his swimming lesson being cancelled, or not having the opportunity to rent a video with me, a weekly ritual. His attention span and focus moved up another notch, and he became very eager to please his aides during his home therapy program. He also began asking his teachers questions when he didn't understand what to do in assignments, without any prompts from his aide. This was also a first.

His reading comprehension and short-term memory improved around this time, and in home therapy, he began recalling the names of characters and settings on his own a half hour after reading the story, and even the following day without prompts. His stool normalized for the first time in six months.

As we had finished his timeline, the following week we began the chronic miasms – hereditary strains of diseases. First came Psora, which was characterized as being the first crack in the deep armour of disease preventing health. I was warned that we might see skin afflictions, aches, pains, and some depression.

The day after finishing the third Psora remedy, Brad came down with a bad cold, cough, and sore throat. He developed blotches on his face and tongue, as well as chapped lips. After 11 days of this we noticed that his coping skills seemed to be improving. He was better able to self-monitor, i.e., to know when he needed a break from a room or activity because his stress and anxiety levels were too high. He was now finally able to comprehend when kids at school were bullying him, even though he didn't know what to do about it.

The following month he took the powders for the second miasm, Tuberculosis, and this caused him to slip back further into the dark again. Once more, his aggression towards me returned. He became more hyperactive, a bit jumpier, and he exhibited less emotional self-regulation both at school and at home. Yet his creative writing abilities seemed to soar at this time. He was writing such imaginative, interesting essays, albeit with some prompts from his school aide, that his teacher was having him go and read them aloud to the principal and other teachers at school.

About a week after taking the Tuberculosis remedies, he had an evening of severe reactions. He crumpled up a sheet of paper with important information on it and threw it in the garbage, glaring at me in defiance, as if he was deliberately trying to hurt me. He would repeatedly pick objects up and look like he was about to hurl them, but then restrain himself at the last minute. At other moments, he would lose all self-restraint and break down and cry, whine, and demand things he knew he couldn't have. He would not go to sleep until midnight. This same behavior repeated itself a couple days later, and then off and on for another several days.

About the same time he had an incident at school where he shouted at a classmate that he wanted to kill him. Another day he broke down and cried when he was at the library with one of his aides. People were staring at him, and he kept asking his aide why, and was then perseverating the rest of the day on the fact that people were looking at him. Each time he would think about it, the tears would come again. It was almost as if he was developing some new self-awareness that people perceived him as odd or strange.

The next miasm was Sycosis, and I was warned that this one could bring on increased hyperactivity, impulsiveness, violence, more intense energy, but at the end of it we should see improved conscious control, improved self-awareness, and the ability to be more present. There was some rather bizarre behavior, such as trying to put his fingers down the garbage disposal while it was running, putting his hands in the toilet bowl, and a great deal of obsessing over past events – not only his misdemeanors but friends who had moved away and aides who had quit working with him and never kept in touch. We also saw an increase in aggression for a week or so, and some increased hyperactivity and inattentiveness, but this was quickly followed by significant improvements in that he became calmer, less anxious, and better behaved at school.

This was June, the end of the school year, and we saw Brad more interested in playing with his peers at recess, instead of always trying to hang around the teachers and talk to them about ceiling fans, hot dog stands, and his other odd interests. He didn't understand all the rules to the games the kids were playing, but he was right in there, trying his best, and they, in turn, were accepting him. It was wonderful to behold!

Academically, there seemed to be some definite improvement as well. He was finally grasping some of the basic Math skills that had eluded him all year. Still far behind his age-appropriate peers, he was starting to catch up. He was doing awesome work in his home therapy program as well. He made some big leaps in his reading comprehension, which had always been a challenge for him. He was able to fill out and correctly answer the worksheets independently that only the week before he required extensive help with.

One evening when his older sister had a friend sleeping over, and Brad was in the bath, he called to me to bring him his housecoat so that he wouldn't have to parade naked down the hall in front of visiting company. While I realize this sounds like a very "normal" thing for a nine-year-old boy, it marked huge progress for Brad. He had never before shown any kind of inhibitions or modesty of this sort. Until very recently, if the doorbell would ring while he was in the bath, he would run, dripping wet and naked to the door to see who was there – behavior one would expect from a two-year-old, but not from a nine-year-old.

Around this time, his stool again turned to explosive diarrhea and the brown water returned. This is mainly a form of discharge of toxins and stress. He also developed a squint in his eyes, which has come and gone ever since. In early July, he seemed to be talking more obsessively again and there was an upswing in his aggression. That same week I gave him Carcinosin, which I was told would likely have little noticeable effect on Brad since he was a *Sulphur* constitutional type and that a *Sulphur* are not much affected by this miasm. Immediately afterwards, however, he dumped his cereal out on the floor, spat in my face, broke a couple objects he threw that evening, and his aggression increased.

Despite these negative behaviors, he was suddenly interested in petting animals and playing appropriately with dogs, whereas he had always been terrified of dogs and had shown no interest in other animals his entire life. At the same time, his use of idiomatic expressions was improving as well.

However, some very bizarre behaviors were starting to emerge. One evening he was repeatedly licking the pages of the book I was reading. He also began playing with himself in the living room, something I had never seen him do before. One evening he urinated on me on purpose. He seemed to become almost more closed-minded, and wouldn't listen to reason.

I learned that these were probably signs that he was ready for the main miasm in autistic children – Syphilis. In mid-July, I gave him the remedies, and immediately he seemed to show vast improvement in every way. With each of the miasms I have seen this immediate response – almost as though he is showing us what he is capable of in the wake of each new remedy. Immediately after taking the *Carcinosin* and *Syphilinum*, we saw big cognitive gains, and even his handwriting looked much more sophisticated and advanced.

After a golden day and a half with the *Syphilinum*, many old behavior problems we hadn't seen in years began to resurface. Brad started picking up discarded cigarette butts and discarded candy from the ground and trying to put them in his mouth again. He was stuffing far too much food into his mouth at mealtime, and the aggression was back full force. Although we had seen all of this in his past, there were two major differences this time. One was that this time he wouldn't listen to reason from anyone, and would just carry on with whatever aberrant behavior he was exhibiting. The other was that it was one thing for a three or four year old to be hitting, biting, scratching, and kicking out of control. But it's a whole other matter when it's a nine-year-old that is five feet tall and very strong.

In response to these new developments, my practitioner sent remedies to help alleviate some of this chthonic realm behavior. The same day Brad deliberately tried to cut himself with a kitchen knife and later on, to break a CD in half. This kind of destructive behavior seemed to cycle in and out of his system, almost like a wave. One minute it was there, the next it was gone again. The following week he was very rigid about anyone touching him and exhibited several anxiety attacks followed by aggression.

This type of behavior continued off and on for the next month, at which time my Heilkünstler suggested giving him *Syphilinum* remedies in LM potency, which seemed to help quite a bit for a few days, and was then followed by the outbreak of another red, raw rash all over his face. The brown, watery diarrhea continued unabated. His obsessive-compulsive behavior had also worsened and he had started reading books in an odd voice, and over accentuating every syllable. For this, I was sent another remedy that seemed to help.

This past month Brad has exhibited a great deal of anxiety, particularly around going to school and being at school. His behavior continues to be quite erratic. Last week we received new remedies for his anxiety to try to address these issues. His gums are sensitive and bleeding again, he just got over another rash on his face, and the diarrhea continues. He is also awake most nights until midnight, often just sitting on his bedroom floor deep in thought for hours on end.

We are now just starting the second round of the miasms. I am awaiting another breakthrough in his condition. It has been a rough couple of months. I also began Heilkunst treatment myself about a year ago, and have found it very beneficial, not only for my own health, but to gain more understanding of what Brad is going through.

In the past year, I, too, along with my son, have gone through tremendous healing. This has helped sustain me by the knowledge that the gains can be painful at times, but are well worth it, and that the only way out is through. Everything else seems to simply palliate in the end.

Jillian's Story

Jillian's parents were concerned about her speech delay, digestive symptoms and constipation, and the diagnosis of PDD (progressive developmental delay). She had developed normally until 18 months, when a loss of language occurred followed by autistic behaviors. There had been some improvement from dietary changes and a number of therapies.

Jillian's treatment began in the Fall of 2003, when she was three and a half, with remedies to remove the negative effects of different antibiotics. Several days after the remedies, Jillian experienced a high fever, and then recovered from her lethargy in three to four days, and there followed some improvement in her condition by the end of the four-week period. Her pupils were less dilated, she was spinning a lot less, she engaged in pretend play with dolls, acting out events from daily life, her hyperactivity and tendency to climb on everything also improved. Her parents stated that this was the "first real improvement" they had seen in her from all the treatments they had previously used.

During the second month, Jillian's tantrums improved, her sleep was "100% better," and she reverted to earlier behaviors, such as hand-slapping and bouncing on a trampoline. For the first time since she had been eight to ten months old, she wanted to play outside. During the next month, she had become toilet-trained and showed greater self-awareness. Overall, her parents stated that she looked much better, and her hair was softer and her dry skin had become less so. She did have some difficulty passing stool.

The second night after the fifth treatment, which was to clear the MMR shock, Jillian threw up, but spoke more spontaneously and increased her pretend play thereafter. Her bowel movements, however, stopped and she only had one unusually large stool one week. A remedy sent to help with the constipation "worked like a miracle." She had a bowel movement the first night and also was no longer crying, which her parents found "remarkable."

After the remedies for the DPT/Hi(b) and Pneumococcocal vaccinations received on the same day, some distinct healing reactions occurred: once a day, Jillian had explosive temper tantrums, screaming when she didn't get what she wanted; her physical sensitivity to noise increased; she became photophobic (a new symptom); and she started taking her clothes off.

On the positive side, she began talking more, and even when she whined it was no longer in a monotone, and involved good language patterns. She was more spontaneous in terms of asking questions, and was overall more expressive, even trying to engage people's eyes to get their attention. Her sleeping patterns were very good, with her sleeping more overall. Her cough of the last few months became more productive and the silver-dollar sized red rings on her skin that had emerged faded by the end of the month. Further improvement, particularly in the tantrums, followed with clearing of the DPT shock.

When her parents also decided to give her a commercial homeopathic formula for candida overgrowth in May, she temporarily regressed in her condition in terms of attentiveness and connection, slept less and began scripting more. We discussed the dosage and also the need to take the next remedies to remove the final vaccination shocks, namely those she had received at birth and shortly thereafter.

Finally, by the end of June she started to improve again – she was calmer, more connected, making eye contact and happier overall. She was even sleeping better again, taking unheard of naps during the day. Her bowel movements returned to normal and her usually swollen abdomen was less distended. A few tantrums recurred by mid-July, but with the next remedies this ended. By August, 2004, she was doing "extremely well."

Parents' Statement

Jillian had a remarkable healing reaction to her first remedy, a course of homeopathic remedies to treat for antiobiotics. She ran a fever of 105F, developed blisters on her lips and slept for almost three straight days.

When her fever subsided, she seemed a lot more calm and connected. Several times we have seen drastic healing reactions, but mainly there have been slow and steady improvements with each remedy. Almost a year after starting sequential homeopathy, Jillian has made huge gains in expressive language. Her eye contact has vastly improved and she now displays affection and laughs appropriately. For us, this emergence of a happier Jillian is the most gratifying thing to come out of her treatment.

Her overall health has also improved. She hasn't had a single ear infection since we started sequential homeopathy. Raised circular rashes that covered her legs, back and stomach have subsided.

We feel that homeopathy, along with one-on-one ABA and floor time therapy, speech, OT, Tomatis, and the Specific Carbohydrate Diet, has played a vital role in our daughter's ongoing recovery.

James' Story

James was about nine when he started treatment with us, being referred by another practitioner. In addition to his diagnosed autistic condition, James also had suffered from epilepsy (which was controlled by drugs), as well as severe headaches. After the first treatment, chosen to stabilize his system as well as to remove the most recent trauma on the timeline (various hospital tests which he found traumatic), James improved in terms of language skills, eye contact, sleep and energy. Overall, his behavior was more appropriate, according to his mother. His headaches also started to improve from the start of treatment.

With the treatment for the shock of the flu on his timeline, James had a return of the frequent drop seizures, which he had had in the past around the flu, but his eye contact improved and his mood became calmer, so much so that when a blood draw was taken he did not react violently as he had in the past.

Following treatment for Prednisone that he had taken in the past, James became more talkative, calmer and much healthier overall. With the next treatment for various accidents and falls, we saw a temporary return of some seizure activity, fears at night and other symptoms from that period, followed by improvements.

His therapist stated that he was doing very well. He no longer banged his head against the wall and was putting more words together. The overall improvement led to some side-effects from the anti-seizure drug until his dosage was lowered. He now began to gain weight and everyone was commenting on how well he looked, how expressive and calm he was and (generally commented) on his greater alertness.

Following treatment for the DPT/Hepatitis B vaccination shock, James experienced significant improvement in his language skills (such as making up his own songs, and using complete sentences), social interaction, and mood, all the while allowing for a continuing reduction in his anti-seizure medication. His neurologist was "amazed" at the changes, according to his mother.

Following treatment for the polio and the Hi(b) vaccination shocks, James saw enough of an improvement in his motor skills that he could work on a computer and was more motivated to do things. By the time we treated for the circumcision, James' bowel movements were browner and firmer, he was more active and could walk much better. When he had an outburst or tantrum, he was able to come back to a calmer level more quickly. He also engaged in more play and teasing.

After removing the DPTP/MMR shock and then the shock from the DPTP/Hi(b)/Hepatitis B vaccinations, James' language skills and social interaction took another significant step forward. He no longer needed naps and had greater stamina. He also started to recall things from the past and discuss them. His speech therapist noticed continued language improvement. Throughout, James had various cleansing or healing reactions involving congestion, tantrums, fever and possibly some seizure activity.

By the end of the summer, James was trying to use long sentences, had great energy, a balanced mood and greater coordination. There remained the DPTP vaccination shock, and also the Tuberculosis vaccination, which he had received on his birth outside of North America. We can expect to see further improvement, and then again when we treat for the inherited weaknesses underlying the autistic condition, which allowed the vaccinations to effectively overwhelm his system.

Parent's Comments

I scanned the article about James and think that it is fairly accurate. The only thing missing is the reaction to the MMR shot. James had a fever and rash on the stomach. He did show some improvements in speech after that treatment too.

Lucas' Story

When Lucas came to us, he was four years old with the diagnosis of "moderate to severe" autism. His timeline was quite familiar, with the various vaccinations (almost 30) common to children in North America. In addition, he had had various rounds of antibiotics for ear infections.

Following his initial treatment with Heilkunst, his sleeping improved significantly and there were also noticeable verbal advancements (more expression and saying people's names, more spontaneity). There did not appear to be any real change after treatment for the DPTP shock, but his fungal/yeast problems worsened and his DAN! doctor put him back on anti-fungals. Nonetheless, there were subtle improvements in verbal skills.

When the MMR shock was treated for, Lucas developed temporary constipation and a skin rash along with further forward movement. Following treatment for the antibiotic shock, Lucas was, "really on solid ground now," according to his mom and this increased with the treatment for the MMR/Chickenpox vaccination shock. He did develop a fairly strong healing reaction, along with some pox, showing the chicken pox virus was being eliminated from the system (often connected with shingles later in life). We are now working on improving his liver function before moving on in the treatment of the vaccination shocks.

Parent's Comments

You may certainly use any info Lucas has given you. He recently finished the MMR/Varicella remedy. Had a week of intestinal issues and spacey behavior. Had a couple of rashes and a few "pox" I am assuming from the varicella. After about a week's time (which has been the last few days) he has come out of this funk and has been very good and clear.

I don't know that I have any fascinatingly dramatic stories for you, just the slow steady picture of a little boy getting better and stronger from the inside out.

Annex A: The Chronic Miasms

A fundamental aspect of Heilkunst is the discovery by its founder, Dr. Samuel Hahnemann, of primary, constant infectious diseases of a chronic nature that can be passed on from one generation to another. These represent archetypal disease forms, out of which emerge the numerous variable, individual diseases.

To the constant infectious forms Dr. Hahnemann gave the name of chronic miasms, as their nature was as constant as those of the acute miasms, like measles or whooping cough. This is part of the tonic side of disease.

The variable forms he termed the chronic diseases, which form part of the pathic side.

"Miasm" is an old medical term for "noxious influence" or "bad air." There are acute miasms, of which the most common are the childhood diseases like measles, mumps, scarlet fever, etc., as well as the well-known infectious diseases such as yellow fever, malaria, cholera, typhoid, and smallpox.

Dr. Hahnemann discovered three chronic miasms: Psora, Sycosis and Syphilis. Later, with the emergence of tuberculosis in the 19th Century, this was also found to be an infectious disease of constant Wesen (essence, or underlying nature). It had been considered part of Psora early on and in some of the books had been initially referred to as pseudo-Psora. Tuberculosis has many features of Psora, but also has aspects of Syphilis. The isolation by Robert Koch, a German scientist, of the tubercular microbe in the late 19th Century confirmed the infectious nature of this miasm.

Later, with the rise of cancer came the discovery by Royal Raymond Rife that cancer too, in its primary form, had an infectious origin. This led to the view that this scourge of mankind was a fifth chronic miasm, sharing elements of Sycosis and Syphilis.

Acute miasms, as with other true acute diseases, have a relatively sudden onset, climax and resolution, and thus are self-limiting. In contrast, the chronic miasms have a slower onset, seldom grow to any climax (although there are periodic flare-ups) and continue until one's death. Their course cannot be prevented, only slowed, by a careful diet and lifestyle, or the absence of stresses. If untreated the prognosis is usually poor and the outcome generally fatal, as we all will tend to die along the same lines, with the same general conditions, from which those in our family tended to die.

The chronic miasms are infectious natural diseases, and each has a characteristic skin lesion. This lesion is the first response of the Living Power in its efforts to evict the disease. If it is unable to do so, the Living Power, in its counter-action, pushes the disturbance, as far as it is able, to the periphery of the organism where it can do the least harm and is visible to the physician so that he can effect a cure.

However, if the natural law of cure is not followed, the treatment only provides temporary relief (palliative) or it suppresses the expression of the disease on the skin and forces the Living Power to set up a line of defense deeper in the organism, affecting the more important (what Hahnemann called "more noble") organs.

Psora

Dr. Hahnemann called the first chronic miasm Psora, from the Hebrew word "tsorat," which has a multitude of meanings, but in this context the sense of "fault, groove, pollution, stigma." It was often applied to leprous manifestations and the great biblical plagues.

Hahnemann was able to trace this disease far back into history, seeing its origins in the reported cases of antiquity of an itch disease, manifesting itself in a skin lesion that was relatively minor, but itchy, particularly if scratched.

Psora is mainly a disease of deficiency at all levels – deficiency of knowledge, thought, assimilation of ideas and nutrition. There are a host of conditions identified by the prefix "hypo" (hypotension, hypochondriasis, hypotrophy) associated with psora. It causes little or no structural change, but much disturbance of functions, feelings and sensations. It seems to involve largely the nervous and reticulo-endocrine systems of the organism.

The psoric state of mind feels it does not have enough (of anything, be it money, food, energy, love, warmth, etc.). You may be familiar with it if you know anyone who had to live through the Great Depression or a war. They may hoard food, toilet paper, rubber bands or twist ties, for no apparent reason other than, "You never know when you may need them." The stereotypical street person illustrates this miasm well, when they are carrying with them every one of their possessions, while wearing virtually all of their clothing, including coats and hats, even in sweltering heat.

If there is psora in your family history, it will manifest, according to Dr. Roger Morrison in his Desktop Guide, as: Abscess. Acne. Allergy. Anxiety. Aphthae. Asthma. Boil. Bronchitis. Colds. Connective tissue disease. Depression. Dermatitis. Eczema. Headache. Insomnia. Otitis media. Pharyngitis. Phobic disorders. Psoriasis. Scabies. Sciatica. Skin ulcers. Upper respiratory infection. (among other conditions)

Sycosis

This chronic miasm is identified by the characteristic small genital warts, which reminded Hahnemann of figs in their shape and texture. The Greek word for fig is sycosis. It originally comes from a gonorrheal infection and leads to various excesses in mind and body function. Here a host of conditions involving the prefix "hyper" are involved (hypertension, hyperactive), as well as inflammatory conditions, various conditions with the suffix "itis" (like sinusitis, vaginitis, urethritis, etc.).

We see in sycosis an excess in mind and tissue, providing the foundation for later tissue degeneration. People who have sycosis are more susceptible to vaccine shock, to the ill-effects of any suppression of morbid discharges (nasal secretions, vaginal discharges, etc.) and to the shock of the surgical removal of various skin manifestations (warts, cysts, fibroids, moles), which can lead to the activation of any latent sycosis.

It seems to involve mainly the blood and circulatory systems, with sycotics being highly susceptible to heart attacks, blood disorders, the ill-effects of blood transfusions, arteriosclerosis, etc. The state of mind is of excess – the sex, drugs and rock-and-roll energy, like Las Vegas at 3:00 a.m., and those who are just getting started at night when others are going to bed.

From Morrison's *Desktop Guide*: Allergy. Angina. Anxiety. Arthritis. Asthma. Behavior disorder. Eczema. Herpes. Hypertension. Interstitial cystitis. Leukorrhea. Manic-depression. Migraine. Otitis. Peptic ulcer. Pulmonary fibrosis. Reiter's syndrome. Sinusitis. Urethritis. Vaginitis. Warts. (among other conditions)

The Sycotic Child

- Extreme extroversion, vitality and energy
- Loud, chattering incessantly, irritating
- Rude and aggressive socially
- Early experience with drugs, sex.
- Sexually precocious behavior (including masturbation, touching of genitals, inappropriate touching of others)
- Hurried behavior, stammering, hyperactivity
- Poor concentration
- Messy by nature
- Meanness and cruelty, frequent fighting, screaming, throwing things, hitting, threats of violence

- Instant gratification, wants things his own way
- Hold deep grudges and resentments; desire for revenge
- Mendacious, jealousy of siblings, selfishness, possessiveness
- Cognitive problems
- Anomalies in gross and fine motor skills
- Short attention span, lack of concentration
- Fears of being alone, of the dark, of large bodies of water, of closed-in spaces
- Night people, restless sleep, nightmares
- Memory weakness

Syphilis

Syphilis is represented by the characteristic genital ulcer and, in general, involves ulcerative conditions. It is marked by tissue destruction and degeneration, involving various conditions marked by the prefix "dys" (such as dystrophy, dystonia). Here we see the corrosive effects of the syphilitic infection in terms of the mind (suicide, serious mental disorders) and the body (ulcers, decay, congenital defects). Most very serious disorders have their roots in this miasm.

The syphilitic patient will lean toward either *self-destruction*, as in bulimia, anorexia, drug or alcohol addictions, obsessive-compulsive disorders (Did I lock the door? Did I lock the door? Did I lock the door? Did I turn off the stove?), and even flesh-eating disease lies in this realm; or *destruction*, including violence toward property or others.

From Morrison's *Desktop Guide*: Abscess. Acne. Alcoholism. Alopecia. Aneurysm. Anxiety. Bone pains. Compulsive disorder. Headache. Insomnia. Leukorrhea. Malignancy. Mouth ulcer. Neuralgia. Psoriasis. Scoliosis. Skin ulcer. Astigmatism. "Growing" pains. (among other conditions)

Tuberculosis

Dr. Hahnemann may have realized later in his life that there was another miasm hidden in Psora. His followers called it "pseudo-Psora" because it had elements of psora, but also of syphilis. This was the term used by homeopaths until later in the 19th Century when tuberculosis emerged as a full-fledged illness in Europe.

The creation of a nosode by J. Compton Burnett in England from the morbid secretion of a tubercular patient (which he named *Baccillinum*), plus the later allopathic discovery of the same infectious agent by Koch, led to Tuberculosis being more closely associated with this newer miasmic discovery. Nebel and Vannier in Europe did more work in identifying the characteristics of Tuberculosis as a chronic miasm.

Tuberculosis is familiar to most of us in its manifestations and appears to have elements of both Psora and Syphilis. One of the keynotes of Tuberculosis is an internal restlessness and degree of consciously-directed destruction.

The person with tuberculosis in the family history has a great desire for change, and it can manifest at any level. They will travel, if possible, to new locales. They may change jobs, change houses, and if those more expensive outlets are not open to them they will change the furniture placement in the house, or paint the walls, or hang new curtains. They cannot even drive to work in the same way every day, because they need the change of route and scenery.

From Morrison's *Desktop Guide*: Adenopathy. Alcoholism. Allergy. Alopecia. Amenorrhea. Arthritis. Asthma. Astigmatism. Autism. Behavior disorder. Bronchitis. Bruxism. Colds. Compulsive disorder. Connective Tissue disease. Croup. Enuresis. Flushes. Headache. Hodgkin's disease. Hyperactivity. Lymphoma. Malignancy. Meningitis. Menopause. Mental retardation. Osteomyelitis. Pneumonia. Respiratory infection. Rheumatoid arthritis. Scoliosis. Sexual disorders. Systemic or discoid lupus. Tinea. Upper respiratory infection. (among other conditions)

The Tubercular Child

- Difficulty in comprehension, poor concentration, averse to mental activity, memory weakness
- Fears of strangers, new situations, dogs, cats, being alone
- Restlessness, intense energy all day, restless sleep
- Grind teeth, toss about in bed
- Love to run, spin and jump
- Strike others
- Worse on waking
- Violent with anger, hitting, biting, throwing fits, striking the head on the ground
- Contrary
- Break things that others value
- Selfish and uncaring about others, property
- Teasing, impish (devil/angel child)

Cancer

The essence of cancer is sensitivity to the world and criticism, and anxiety for others and events generally. It shares some noteworthy features of Tuberculosis, such as hair on the spine, blue sclerae, genupectoral sleep position and the desire for travel. There are also links to Sycosis – hyperactivity in children, increased sexual desire, amelioration by the ocean, desire for salt, sweets and fats, and insomnia.

Carcinosin is fastidious and worse from consolation. It desires chocolate and has a love of dancing. It is exhilarated in thunderstorms. It has a strong connection with the constitutional remedy *Silicea* and also to *Natrum mur*. The essence of cancer is resignation, a loss of the self, living for others and not realizing their own destiny.

It is also a great remedy for opposites. There can be great love or desire, then intense hate or aversion.

The child can have high fevers or no childhood fevers. They have a magnetic energy and attraction. The sexual desire of the cancer type is high.

From Morrison's *Desktop Guide*: Abscess. Acne. Allergy. Asthma. Chronic fatigue syndrome. Colitis. Constipation. Cough. Developmental delay. Diabetes. Dysmenorrhea. Headache. Immune deficiency. Insomnia. Moles. Nevi. Ovarian cyst. Premenstrual syndrome. Rectal prolapse. Respiratory illness. Sinusitis. Tics. (among other conditions).

We have discovered, based on close observation of our cases, that most people have most of the chronic miasms through inheritance. We also have the discovery of a particular order of appearance of these miasms during treatment. This particular order, called the law of succession of forces by its discoverer, Dr. Elmiger of Switzerland, adds to the sequence of treatment that Hahnemann laid down in his writings.

Annex B: The Chthonic Realm

This is the realm of fear, which Dr. Hahnemann called our "deepest disease." Anxiety is a necessary condition of man in his natural state. However, when we are living in disease, the alterations created in our inner knowing turn anxiety into fear.

We are born into a state of "sin," that is, simply a division or separation from our inner knowing (the word for sin in Greek is a technical term meaning "to miss the mark" as in the bull's eye in archery), and as our intellect, our awareness of self emerges, so does our separation from our inner knowing (wisdom). What we have lost in wisdom over the centuries, we have gained in individual liberty and sense of self as unique entities.

However, because of disease we have filled our growing state of ignorance of the world with beliefs that block a return to our wisdom. This return must not be simply a return to our previous state, but the creation of a new state of conscious knowing that integrates our inner wisdom (intuition, imagination, inspiration) with our awareness of self and world, a state of super-consciousness that is founded on this integration of sense and super-sense within us.

Instead of the constant strife within between instinct and intellect, we need to have a form of true reason that is the basis of a true science of self and non-self. This true science is one that will finally cut through the Gordian knot of Western philosophy (false polarity between spirit and matter) and free us from the tyranny of both materialism and mysticism.

We have been able to discover and map the chthonic realm, thanks to the principles of Heilkunst and the clinical experiences provided by the cases we have treated. Our own process of discovery has been like the era of discovery of the world by Western explorers, and every case has been like an initial voyage, each time taking us further and deeper into the unknown, expanding our map of the known, leaving the familiar coastline of our rational world and venturing into the oceanic unknown, full of mythical monsters and dangers, some real, and many illusory.

While we have been able to circumnavigate the globe, many areas remain uncharted and vague, waiting for future expeditions to shed light and fill in the map of our conscious understanding. What we have to date is the broad outline of the chthonic realm and an approach to treatment that is grounded in natural law.

Our research has revealed that there is a dual stream, each of which exists within us, but one of which may be more dominant. One of the streams, which we term the "hot stream," is more overt and visible in its expression, with external manifestations of fear. The other is less visible, and we term it the "cold stream." It expresses itself more by the fear going inward.

For each of the streams, there seem to be four phases and four medicines that address them. What follows below is a summary of the state of mind and condition of each remedy.

Hot Stream

***Stramonium*:** When someone needs *Stramonium* they feel alone, helpless and forsaken in a world that feels overwhelmingly terrifying and dangerous, and their behavior will reflect that fear. Their fears may be exacerbated in the dark and at night, when they may feel more vulnerable, and they may be clingy and needy during the night or at bedtime, or fearful to be alone in a room without a nightlight on or in the company of a parent.

They may become destructive of their clothes and may strike out, and act with violence and fear, all with a sense of self-preservation and defensiveness. In an extreme state the level of violence escalates, and it can be turned inward or outward, with shrieking, biting, screaming, tearing and even cursing. Someone needing *Stram* may have a fear of animals, particularly dogs (fearing the dogs will attack them), and worse still may be black dogs. They also can have fears of tunnels or other enclosed places, as well as deep water and mirrors.

Stram symptoms will arise from a sudden shock, blow to the head, birth injuries, an intense fright, or with a very high fever and/or neurological damage, often seen post-vaccination.

***Hyoscyamus*:** The fears and energy of *Hyoscyamus* manifest after a shock that causes them to behave as if they have lost all trust, faith, safety and security in those who are supposed to bc there to love and protect them. They are so terrified of being alone (or *feeling* deserted) that they draw attention to themselves, almost in a manic way, with exaggerated behaviors, from joking and laughing, acting silly, being loquacious and immature, to violence, striking, and acting in shamelessly sexually provocative ways. They will expose themselves or fondle their genitals, and speak or joke in lewd ways. Their state is less intensely destructive than that of *Stram*.

In the back of their minds, those needing *Hyos* feel that if they do not keep the attention of those they love, need or depend upon, they will lose them, and so they will show extreme behaviors out of this fear.

They also have a more internal state, muttering to themselves or talking with people who are not there. They can obsess, usually over small and simple things, and repeat the same tasks over and over and over again. They may lose control of urination and defecation, and may be fine sitting in it, or spending hours playing with their stool. People needing *Hyos* also will pick at things, like dust particles in the air, or specks on their clothing. They have symptoms on hearing running water, and may urinate or defecate involuntarily, or dread hearing running water and react with fear.

***Belladonna*:** The energy around *Belladonna* is intense! It is acute, hot and obvious. The person needing *Bell* can be happy, dancing, singing and apparently fine one minute, then react with an intense fear, as if there is some massive threat to their life. They may feel the need to run, to escape, to rage, all because they feel they need to save themselves from this imminent danger.

They may be extremely sensitive to noise, light and jarring and avoid bright and noisy places. They do not avoid company, but the stimulation that can come from being with people can be overwhelming for them. The intensity of *Bell* is a keynote – red, hot, with violent impulses. They may want to tear their clothes, or be tempted to bite or pull someone's hair. They have a fear of animals in general, and dogs more specifically.

There can be a delirious state where the person laughs at imaginary things that they see, they can strike out at imaginary objects, knock their head against the wall, or they may sit quietly and break small sticks repeatedly. They may bark or growl like a dog, and feel compelled to touch everything in the room.

The origin of the *Bell* state can come from strong fevers, injuries to the head and suppression of eruptions.

***Veratrum album*:** *Veratrum* is busy. There is much less violence than in the other hot stream chthonic remedies, but there is a great deal of industriousness. They are not destructive, but those needing *Verat* seem to have an endless supply of energy (exhausting for parents), which they use to ceaselessly draw, sing, clean, or do perseverative behaviors and repetitious things like stack CDs, stimming behavior with calculators, etc. This is a very intense remedy, but more in terms of the energy they expend daily than in any violent or destructive way.

Another side of *Verat* is a melancholy, with an air of superiority and righteousness, which may or may not have religious overtones. They may feel that they are sane and the rest of us are insane; they may hold themselves above the rules, which don't apply to them. They can look at their parents as if the demands placed on mere commoners in no way could apply to them, with their elevated stature. It is as if their ego is very fragile and they have to protect themselves by withdrawing from the ordinary world.

Some keynotes of *Verat* are a desire for eating ice and other cold things, and fruit, particularly acidic fruits, and salt. They can have a physical coldness as well, feeling cold to the touch. They are prone to sudden diarrhea that seems to be forcibly ejected from the body, and can have vomiting and diarrhea concurrently.

Cold Stream

***Baryta carb*:** Immaturity is a keynote of *Baryta carb*, and it can be seen on any level, from physical immaturity and slow development of single body parts, to an immature dependence on others for emotional support. They may be quite capable intellectually, performing well in school, but are socially shy and insecure, unable to feel safe without a strong connection with those they feel offer protection. They are also disconnected in terms of their emotions, and are not able to make a connection between what emotions would feel like and how to express them. They can be terrified that something bad will happen to those upon whom they depend.

Those needing *Bar-c* may have the inability to retain food or to swallow solid foods. They can sit and brood in a corner in their house for hours, and experience panic when asked to go out into the world. They can have a fear of strangers and of new situations, and may startle easily and be frightened of loud noises. They cannot conceive of pleasure, and are so dependent and immature that they don't want to socialize or mix with those outside their safety net.

***Arnica*:** The symptoms of *Arnica* come from a very deep, traumatic assault on the individual either mentally, emotionally or physically, and as a result they are seriously wounded, "bruised," and in pain, on one level or another. This leaves them with the sense that the world is unsafe and painful, that they need to protect themselves from all contact with people or situations that could hurt them again.

They may be irritable, angry, argumentative and unapproachable, but this behavior serves them by ensuring no one comes too close. They may want something and then, once it is given, push it away, unable to know what it is they truly want and don't want.

Another side of *Arn* is where the person is passive, sensitive and touchy. They may want to be left alone, not talk with anyone and avoid human contact, and may be upset with consolation and conversation, and want to be more quiet and process things internally.

***Helleborus*:** In the Helleborus state there is *so* much pain that the person seeks to shut himself off from the world completely. It is as if the physical body is there, but there is no one at home inside. His eyes are fine, but he doesn't see. His ears are okay, but he does not hear. He may take a long time before responding to a question. He is not able to make decisions for himself, not even when asked what he'd like to eat.

The faces of those needing *Hell* may lack expression, and they may look bewildered and confused. They may sit and moan, and often do have quite a vivid imagination with a lot of activity in their mind, but it's just not able to be expressed. They also may roll their head, from side to side, as in encephalitis.

Hell is sometimes better with a violent shock, as if it takes something dramatic to penetrate their shut down state of mind. A loud shout or yell may get a response, and they may slap or hit themselves, perhaps for the stimulation it brings and to maintain a sense of connection.

***Bufo*:** The keynote of *Bufo* is a strong sexual element. This can show up in the form of solitary intellectual or mental pursuits, what can be referred to as mental masturbation, or actual physical masturbation. The person needing *Bufo* is immature, childish and highly sexual. There is no self-control over their instinctual desires, whether they are for eating or physical/sexual stimulation (without shame) or sitting alone in the basement on the computer for hours on end. They need their desires to be fulfilled and they do not understand why they would have to postpone them to a more appropriate time or place, or to limit them in any way.

They may have childish laughter and an immature sense of humor, and have a fear of animals. They may strike out, or be destructive, but more often they are seen as loners who want to remain in solitude to stimulate themselves one way or another. They may appear to be larger and more fleshy physically than other types, and are known for a dull look on their faces with their tongues protruding from thicker lips.

Annex C: Dynamic Pharmacy

Similars and Opposites

The nature of a medicine lies in its very capacity to negatively affect the living organism at a dynamic level. In a very real sense all medicines must be poisons, although some of them may have a low toxicity in their crude state, or we may have become accustomed to their effects through long usage. This is the case with common salt *(Natrum muriaticum)* or various spices such as red pepper (*Capsicum*). However, *all* have the ability to affect our Dynamis.

When medicine is used on a false basis, as is the case, by and large, in allopathic medicine ("allo" means that it operates on no principle of nature), it may also have a seeming positive effect, in terms of temporary relief of some of a patient's symptoms. However, this is achieved only through suppressing the expression of the underlying disease in the patient.

This temporary relief is seen as desirable, though the negative effects of a medicine are seen as unwanted (referred to as "adverse effects" or more commonly as "side effects"). These unwanted effects are, in reality, the disease effects of that medicine on the patient. That is, each medicinal substance has the potential to engender a medicinal disease in a patient. It is this power to affect the generative aspect of the Living Power of a living being that makes them medicines in the first place.

When a medicine is used on the basis of the correct principle, that is the curative law of similars, then it has a true positive or therapeutic affect.

The Importance of Dose

However, the issue of dose is almost as important as the selection of the remedy on the basis of the correct principle. If the dose is not correctly chosen, then there also remains a potential negative effect. As Dr. Hahnemann, the founder of Heilkunst, stated:

> §275.1. The appropriateness of a medicine for a given case of disease does not rest alone on its apt homeopathic selection, but just as well on the requisite, correct size or, rather smallness of its dosage.
>
> §275.2. If an all too strong dose is given (for the present disease state) of even a completely homeopathically chosen medicine, so must it nevertheless, notwithstanding the beneficence of its nature in itself, certainly inflict damage due to its size and the here unnecessary, overly strong impression which it makes on the Living Power by virtue of its resonant homeopathic action throughout precisely those most sensitive parts of the organism already attacked most by the natural disease.
>
> §276.1. For this reason a medicine, even if it was homeopathically appropriate to the disease case, does damage in every dose that is too large, and in strong doses all the more, the greater the homeopathicity and the higher the potency that was selected, and to be sure, far more than every equally large dose of an unhomeopathic (allopathic) medicine bearing no relation to the disease state.

Suppression and Iatrogenesis vs. Cure

Medicines truly are a two-edged sword. In the hands of allopathy, the sword causes damage in both directions:

- suppression of the original disease, which only serves to drive it deeper into the organism and weaken the resistance, creating chronic, protracted problems, and
- the engendering of a new, medicinal disease in the patient, that must now be treated.

In the hands of the true physician (Heilkünstler, that is, one who practices the system of medicine called Heilkunst), the "sword" is able to cure without causing any damage. This is partly because of the manner in which medicines are prepared (highly diluted and shaken so that they act energetically or dynamically) and the use of the optimal dose (just enough to cure and no more).

In keeping with the medical approach of his time, Dr. Hahnemann initially used mainly crude doses applied on the basis of the law of similars. He was able to achieve curative results, but he noticed that some medicinal disease effects also occurred. He sought continually to *reduce* the dose in order to lessen the adverse effects of the medicine, while still retaining some positive, therapeutic effect.

In the thinking of his day, still prevalent today, the effect of a medicine was ascribed to the chemical constituents of the crude, material substance.

Being a chemist, Dr. Hahnemann was well aware of this. However, his concern for his patients and his sensitivity to the disease effects of medicines led him to begin to dilute the usual fairly material dose (usually in grams or the equivalent of milligrams) of such poisons as arsenic, mercury, and plant poisons such as *Aconite* (Monkshood), *Belladonna* (Deadly Nightshade), *Hyosycamus* (Henbane), *Helleborus* (Black Hellebore), *Veratrum album* (White Hellebore), *Conium* (Hemlock), etc. Even before he formally founded his new system of medicine, he departed from the medical conventions of his day and used medicines in quite small doses.

When Dr. Hahnemann first began to apply the law of similars as the principle for medicine in his cases after around 1790, he still used these material, if relatively small, doses in treatment. However, he noticed that this caused an initial apparent aggravation of the patient's symptoms as the similar medicine caused a temporary artificial disease in the patient similar, but not identical, to the natural disease of the patient.

He called this the "homeopathic aggravation." The more similar the remedy, the more there was a risk of this homeopathic aggravation, such that the issue of dose became very important. Indeed, as Dr. Hahnemann knew, the law of similars had been known by physicians in the past but had been abandoned because it was too dangerous in crude doses (as is still the case in conventional vaccinations). Dr. Hahnemann's work in adjusting the dose provided a new lease on this ancient principle.

So he began a gradual process, over two decades, of reducing the dose. Dr. Hahnemann proceeded slowly, as he was still caught up in the material notion of dose that governed science and medicine. However, he also had a growing awareness that there was an energetic or dynamic element involved in the process of remediation (heilen). The care with which he proceeded indicates that he was concerned about establishing a firm foundation for any dosage approach for his new medical system.

> 4.1 What would they have risked had they straight away followed my directions in the beginning, and had made use of just these small doses from the very first? Could anything worse have happened than that these doses might not have helped? They surely could do no harm! But in their injudicious, self-willed application of large doses for homeopathic application they only traversed once again that roundabout road to reach the truth, so dangerous to their patients, which I myself had already in trembling but successfully passed over so as to spare them this trouble; and if they really desired to cure, they were nevertheless

at last compelled to arrive at the only true goal, after having inflicted much mischief and wasted a goodly part of their life. All this I had already long before laid before them faithfully and frankly, and well-grounded.

Dilution and Potentisation

Let's first look at the standardization that Dr. Hahnemann developed over time for his medicines.

Hahnemann began to take one drop or one grain (almost a poppy seed-sized amount) of a given substance and dilute it in a given quantity of water, usually 100, 200 or 300 drops of water/alcohol. He later standardized this to 99 drops of water and alcohol solution (usually an 80%:20% mixture).

He also took pains to thoroughly agitate the resulting solution, by a process he called succussion.

Succussion involved, in Hahnemann's case, taking the small glass vial of the solution and shaking it by a quick flick of the arm in a downward motion, or by brisk stirring. Later he advised to strike the vial of the solution onto a firm, but still flexible surface, such as a leather-bound book. This process clearly mixed the solution so that the single drop was now spread throughout the new solution.

What he discovered was that this vigorous mixing, what he referred to also as "intimate" mixing, released a spirit-like energy within the crude substance that often was not noticeable in its crude form, such as in the case of *Lycopodium* seeds (club moss) or salt. And he discovered that medicines had a Wesen, or a dynamic aspect.

The mix of one drop of herbal mother tincture (the concentrate from the soaking of the plant – either the whole plant, or the leaves, roots, bark or fruit alone) and 99 drops of water/alcohol mix gave a solution of 100 drops. The concentration of the medicine in such a solution was then 1/100 or 10^{-2}.

Let's look at how this process of sequential dilution works:

First, we begin, in the case of a plant or soluble mineral, such as a salt, with the stock solution. For an herb, this is referred to as the Mother Tincture (MT), or Tincture mère in French (TM).

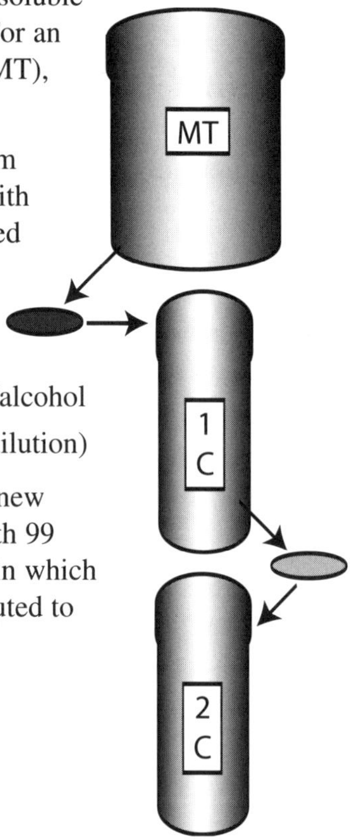

Next, Dr. Hahnemann took one drop from this stock solution and placed it in a glass vial with 99 drops of pure water/alcohol. He then succussed this solution (anywhere from 10-100 times), and that he
named 1C.

1 drop medicine to 99 drops of water/alcohol
= 1/100 or 10^{-2} = 1C (C is for centesimal dilution)

If we then take, in turn, one drop of the new solution (1C) and add it again to another vial with 99 drops of water/alcohol, we now have a solution in which the original substance from the MT has been diluted to 1/1000 or 10^{-4}.

This is now labeled as a 2C solution.

1 drop of 1C solution to 99 drops of
water/alcohol = 1/10000 or 10^{-4} = 2C

This process can be continued many times using the same approach. Dr. Hahnemann worked mainly with the dilutions up to 30C by 1816. By the time of his death, he had apparently used as high as a 1M (or 1000C).

Korsakov Method

Dr. Korsakoff (or Korsakov, as the spelling varies) also, for practical reasons, developed a new method of producing dilutions. Whereas Hahnemann used a new vial for each dilution, Korsakoff simply emptied the vial in use and added to it 99 parts of water/alcohol to produce the next dilution. Observation had convinced him that at least one drop's equivalent of the solution remained in the vial when it was emptied. Thus, adding the 99 drops of water/alcohol to the same vial when "empty" had the same effect as taking a drop of the solution and putting it in a new vial with 99 drops of water/alcohol.

This method was less expensive and time-consuming than Hahnemann's more precise and methodical approach, and worked particularly well in the higher potencies. For example, to produce a 200C potency by Hahnemann's method would require 200 vials, whereas this could be done with only one vial using the Korsakoff method. The latter also lends itself better to mechanization.

Thus, the Korsakoff method is generally the one most used today, particularly and almost exclusively in the higher potencies (above 200C). To distinguish the two methods, the potencies made using the Hahnemannian approach are designated with an H (e.g., 3CH) and the potencies made by the Korsakoff method have the designation K (200CK or 200K).

Trituration

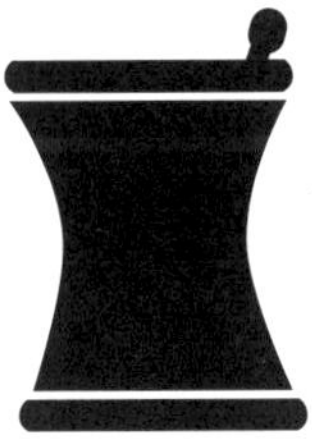

Dr. Hahnemann also began, around 1816, to refer to his dilutions as "potencies" or "power developments." Although he had been aware since around 1800 that the medicines acted dynamically, and not materially, it seems that he became more conscious of that reality when he discovered the ability to take substances that were innocuous in their crude state (such as salt, charcoal, lycopodium, silica, lime, etc.) and render them effective through prolonged trituration. (Haehl, Vol. I, p. 317) The detailed directions for trituration were first given to the public with the publication of the first edition of Hahnemann's *Chronic Diseases* (1828, Vol. II) and in the second edition (Vol. I, p. 182).

Essentially, one part of the original substance (dry plants, sapless native plants, metals, minerals and all other insoluble substances) is mixed with 99 parts of milk sugar (lactose) and ground for an hour using a mortar and pestle. This is called the 1st trituration. One part of this is then taken and ground for an hour with another 99 parts of lactose to produce the 2nd trituration. Only when he reached the 3rd trituration did Dr. Hahnemann find that the substance could be dissolved in liquid and then further diluted using the method above.

Decimal Scale

Later, homeopaths developed a dilution on a decimal scale for the lower potencies. Here, one drop of mother tincture is diluted in 9 drops of water/alcohol giving a 1X or 1D potency. The "D" stands for "decimal." This scale is mainly used in Europe.

Annex D: Homeopathy and Heilkunst

Homeopathy, or *homeopathic* (as in "homeopathic philosophy"), is generally taken to refer to the system of medicine that Dr. Samuel Hahnemann established between about 1790 and his death in 1843, as well as its subsequent practice around the world. However, homeopathy is only one part of a much broader system of medicine founded by Dr. Hahnemann, which he termed *Heilkunst.*

As can be seen from the body of this book, Heilkunst encompasses a wide range of approaches, and is essentially a framework of principles derived from natural law that direct how and when a given therapy or approach, including homeopathy, should be correctly and effectively used and applied.

Homeopathy, in its strict sense, refers only to that use of the natural law of cure, the law of similars as it is applied in variable, mostly natural diseases, which manifest themselves in changes in feelings, functions and sensations, or the pathology (suffering) of an individual.

Homeopathic as applied to medicines is another term that is widely misused. It is popularly taken to mean any substance that has been diluted and succussed. However, its correct meaning is a substance, whether crude or potentized, that is chosen on the basis of the symptoms of the disease using the law of similars. No substance is homeopathic until it is applied successfully in this manner.

An example of this is one of the remedies that might be used for symptoms of hayfever – *Allium cepa* is made from a red onion, and its similar symptoms might include watery, burning red eyes and a runny nose. But if you are in a hyperalert state of mind, your mind too busy to allow you to fall asleep, according to the law of similars you could use a small bit of coffee, in its crude form, to help you to calm your mind enough to relax and fall asleep. In both of these examples, the substances (whether potentized or not) acted homeopathically.

Annex E: Definition of Autistic Condition

From the Diagnostic and Statistical Manual of Mental Disorders, Fourth Edition (DSM IV):

Diagnostic Criteria for 299.00 Autistic Disorder

A. A total of six (or more) items from (1), (2), and (3), with at least two from (1), and one each from (2) and (3)

(1) Qualitative impairment in social interaction, as manifested by at least two of the following:

a) Marked impairments in the use of multiple nonverbal behavior such as eye-to-eye gaze, facial expression, body posture, and gestures to regulate social interaction.

b) Failure to develop peer relationships appropriate to developmental level.

c) A lack of spontaneous seeking to share enjoyment, interests, or achievements with other people, (e.g., by a lack of showing, bringing, or pointing out objects of interest to other people).

d) Lack of social or emotional reciprocity. Note: in the description, it gives the following as examples: not actively participating in simple social play or games, preferring solitary activities, or involving others in activities only as tools or "mechanical" aids.

(2) Qualitative impairments in communication as manifested by at least one of the following:

a) Delay in, or total lack of, the development of spoken language (not accompanied by an attempt to compensate through alternative modes of communication such as gesture or mime).

b) In individuals with adequate speech, marked impairment in the ability to initiate or sustain a conversation with others.

c) Stereotyped and repetitive use of language of idiosyncratic language.

d) Lack of varied, spontaneous make-believe play or social imitative play appropriate to developmental level.

(3) Restricted repetitive and stereotyped patterns of behavior, interests and activities, as manifested by at least two of the following:

a) Encompassing preoccupation with one or more stereotyped and restricted patterns of interest that is abnormal either in intensity or focus.

b) Apparently inflexible adherence to specific, nonfunctional routines or rituals.

c) Stereotyped and repetitive motor mannerisms (e.g., hand or finger flapping or twisting, or complex whole-body movements).

d) Persistent preoccupation with parts of objects.

B. Delays or abnormal functioning in at least one of the following areas, with onset prior to age 3 years:

(1) social interaction

(2) language as used in social communication

(3) symbolic or imaginative play

C. The disturbance is not better accounted for by Rett's Disorder or Childhood Disintegrative Disorder.

Autism and Pervasive Developmental Disorder

From the Autism Society of America (www.autism-society.org)

Diagnosing Autism, PDD, or Asperger's Disorder

The term "PDD" is widely used by professionals to refer to children with autism and related disorders; however, there is a great deal of disagreement and confusion among professionals concerning the PDD label. Diagnosis of PDD, Autism, or any other developmental disability, is based upon the Diagnostic and Statistical Manual of Mental Disorders - Fourth Edition (DSM-IV), published by the American Psychiatric Association, Washington D.C., 1994, the main diagnostic reference of Mental Health professionals in the United States of America.

According to the DSM-IV, the term "PDD" is not a specific diagnosis, but an umbrella term under which the following specific diagnoses are defined:

- Autistic Disorder
- Rett's Disorder
- Childhood Disintegrative Disorder
- Asperger's Disorder
- Pervasive Developmental Disorder Not Otherwise Specified (PDD-NOS)

Diagnostic labels are used to indicate commonalities among individuals. The diagnosis of autism indicates the existence of qualitative impairments in communication, social skills, and range of interests and activities. As no medical tests can be performed to indicate the presence of autism or any other PDD, the diagnosis is based upon the presence or absence of specific behaviors. For example, a child may be diagnosed as having PDD-NOS if he or she has some behaviors that are seen in autism, but does not meet the full criteria for having autism. Most importantly, whether a child is diagnosed with PDD, PDD-NOS, or autism, his or her treatment will be similar.

Vaccinations: The Overlooked Factors

by Bernard Rimland, Ph.D.
Autism Research Institute
4182 Adams Avenue
San Diego, CA 92116

Vaccinations, like motherhood and apple pie, have long been regarded as taboo topics, beyond criticism. No more. The publication in The Lancet of the article by Andrew Wakefield and associates, providing a well-documented mechanism for the long suspected role of MMR vaccines in causing autism, has raised an international furor.

I began to suspect a link between the DPT vaccination and autism as early as in the mid 1960s, based on letters from and interviews with many parents. Our Form E-3 parent questionnaire, dating from 1967, asked parents about their children's reaction to the DPT shot. H. L. Coulter and B. L. Fisher state, in their excellent book, DPT: Shot in the Dark (1985), "The phenomenon of early infantile autism was first observed and discussed by physicians in the early 1940s, a few years after the pertussis vaccine became more widely used in the United States... The parallel to certain areas of pertussis vaccine damage is striking" (p. 123).

Readers of the Autism Research Review International (ARRI) are well aware of the autism-vaccine controversy (see ARRI 10/4, 10/1, 9/3, 9/2, 9/1, 6/3), but until now the mass media have been kept largely in the dark. In Britain, where there has been an epidemic of autism, with hundreds of families registering for projected class-action law suits, some newspapers have been devoting half-page or larger articles to the controversy.

Dr. Wakefield and his courageous collaborators have endured a torrent of criticism and abuse from those dedicated to silencing anyone challenging the sacred-cow status of vaccines. The fact is, vaccines are not nearly as safe, nor anywhere near as effective, as vaccination proponents claim.

Dr. Wakefield's opponents argue, quite speciously, that he is confusing association with causation, and that the autism link may be merely "coincidental."

I find it doubly ironic that the vaccine advocates accuse Wakefield of this elementary error in logic. That very argument was used just as wrongly - against vaccinations - by the opponents of Edward Jenner when he introduced vaccination to Europe. (It was used earlier in Asia.) Jenner's observation that milkmaids exposed to pox-infected cows developed a resistance to smallpox was attributed to coincidence. Fortunately for today's vaccine proponents, Jenner's critics did not succeed in dismissing his observations as merely "coincidence."

The second irony is that the critics who accuse Dr. Wakefield of confusing association with causation are guilty of doing that very thing - deliberately, not mistakenly - while trying to influence public policy, by claiming that vaccines cause steep declines in the incidence of disease when there is good evidence that the decline was often due to other factors, that is, to coincidence.

In their reply to Wakefield's article, "Vaccine adverse effects: causal or coincidental?" R.T. Chen and F. DeStephano (Lancet 2/28/98) present a table implying that the incidence of a number of diseases was enormously reduced by vaccinations. In fact, judging from data presented by Neil Z. Miller in his book *Vaccines, are They Safe and Effective?,* the reductions Chen and DeStephano cite are often coincidental rather than causal. In the case of measles, the death rate did drop precipitously over a period of four decades, but the death rate fell 95% before the measles vaccine was introduced! In the case of polio, the death rate had dropped 60% from its peak in the 1920s and '30s before the vaccines arrived in the 1950s. There is considerable evidence that the claims of benefit for other vaccines (e.g., pertussis, tetanus) are also greatly inflated.

There is an enormous amount of credible evidence that vaccines can and do cause harm. In response to what was seen as a cause-and-effect relationship with sudden infant death syndrome (SIDS), the Japanese government, in 1979, ordered the postponement of routine DPT shots until after the age of two. "SIDS has virtually disappeared from Japan" (Neil Z. Miller, *Immunization, Theory vs. Reality* [1996].) In an article titled, "The Dark Side of Immunizations?," Science News (November 22, 1997) reported findings by scientists implicating the rise in diabetes and asthma to vaccines, and these allegations are just the tip of a very large iceberg. (The medical establishment's ferocious defense of vaccines as irrefutably safe and beneficial somehow reminds me of the Titanic.)

I am not saying that vaccinations are without value. I am saying that their benefits have been overstated, and their dangers dismissed much too carelessly.

QUESTIONS.

The Black Death is estimated to have killed one third of the population of Europe before it subsided. Why did it subside? Largely because the immune system is a marvelously adaptable instrument which learned, naturally, how to cope with the plague.

Interesting though it is that one out of three died of the plague, it is even more interesting that two out of three lived. Why?

Although the headlines alarmed us all when some people died as a result of the swine flu vaccine and some people died when exposed to Legionnaire's disease, it is even more interesting that most people survived. Why? Why are some children injured by MMR shots and others not?

The answer is that people are very different, in many ways. Part of the difference is genetic. Another part is environmental.

We can't do much about the genetic part right now, but we can do a lot about each person's susceptibility to disease, including vaccine-induced disease, by dealing intelligently with the environment.

TOXIC EXPOSURE. It is no secret that our environment is loaded with toxins, many of which greatly impair not only the brain but also the immune system. Lead, mercury, pesticides, and solvents all can create havoc with the immune system. There is of course a huge literature on this topic. Two excellent recent books are: *Our Toxic World: Who is Looking After our Kids* by H. E. Buttram, M.D., and Richard Piccolo (1996), and *Is This Your Child's World?* by Doris Rapp, M.D. (1997).

NUTRITION. In my view, the most important and by far the most feasible approach to preventing damage by toxins of all kinds, including the toxins in vaccines (vaccines contain mercury, aluminum and formaldehyde, in addition to germs) is to help the child's developing, immature immune system by providing generous amounts of the nutrients the body needs if it is going to be able to protect itself from a dangerous, toxin-laden world.

In his book *Every Second Child* (1981), Archie Kalokerinos, an Australian physician, tells us that the death rate among the aborigine children he was assigned to help was an astounding 50%! His investigation showed these deaths to be associated with vaccinations, and he found the children's diets to be severely deficient in vitamin C. By merely administering vitamin C (100 mg per month of age), he dropped the death rate to nearly zero.

In my view, and in the view of many others who have studied these problems, every mother-to-be, starting well before conception, should be taking significant (several grams a day, at least) amounts of vitamin C, and every child should also be given supplements—especially in view of the stress on the immune system imposed by vaccines.

But vitamin C is by no means the only nutrient that should be supplemented if the immune system is to develop and function effectively. Nutrients known to be effective in autism, vitamin B6 and DMG, have been shown in laboratory studies to enhance immune function. The minerals zinc and selenium, both implicated in many cases of autism, are critical in immune function.

Nutrition is the single most important determinant of immune function, according to world authority R. K. Chandra, who specifically mentions zinc, selenium, iron, copper, vitamins A, C, E, B6, and folic acid.

The message is very clear: mothers should take a high quality, broad-spectrum vitamin and mineral supplement before conception, and during pregnancy and lactation. And every child should also be getting extra nutrients through mother's milk or along with food, if the immune system is to develop properly. The cost of not doing so may be very high.

Number of Autistic Children Ages 6-21 Served Under IDEA, Part B

During the 2001-02 School Year

STATE	1992-1993	1999-2000	2001-2002
Alabama	68	670	904
Alaska	8	165	223
Arizona	199	897	1,348
Arkansas	30	560	774
California	1,605	8,376	13,257
Colorado	14	350	538
Connecticut	164	1,032	1,470
Delaware	15	248	294
District of Columbia	0	65	144
Florida	582	3,114	4,328
Georgia	262	1,602	2,462
Hawaii	52	198	380
Idaho	39	239	356
Illinois	5	2,435	3,802
Indiana	273	2,080	3,262
Iowa	67	543	554
Kansas	74	471	743
Kentucky	38	739	1,022
Louisiana	409	1,032	1,297

Maine	**37**	**358**	**552**
Maryland	**28**	**1,551**	**2,396**
Massachusetts	**493**	**543**	**2,681**
Michigan	**288**	**3,449**	**7,719**
Minnesota	**296**	**1,958**	**3,270**
Mississippi	**0**	**333**	**461**
Missouri	**336**	**1,361**	**1,953**
Montana	**20**	**127**	**197**
Nebraska	**4**	**289**	**415**
Nevada	**5**	**273**	**518**
New Hampshire	**0**	**268**	**404**
New Jersey	**446**	**2,378**	**3,526**
New Mexico	**16**	**193**	**265**
New York	**1,648**	**4,951**	**7,023**
North Carolina	**786**	**2,391**	**3,095**
North Dakota	**9**	**98**	**144**
Ohio	**22**	**1,574**	**3,057**
Oklahoma	**31**	**547**	**785**
Oregon	**37**	**2,218**	**2,847**
Pennsylvania	**346**	**2,707**	**3,969**
Puerto Rico	**266**	**408**	**518**
Rhode Island	**19**	**238**	**384**
South Carolina	**141**	**717**	**1,012**
South Dakota	**36**	**168**	**250**

Tennessee	**304**	**819**	**1,103**
Texas	**1,444**	**5,134**	**7,099**
Utah	**105**	**472**	**723**
Vermont	**6**	**160**	**248**
Virginia	**539**	**1,714**	**2,365**
Washington	**476**	**1,376**	**1,972**
West Virginia	**101**	**262**	**374**
Wisconsin	**18**	**1,445**	**2,247**
Wyoming	**15**	**83**	**117**
Total	**12,222**	**65,396**	**100,847**

Data based on the December 1, 2001 count, updated as of August 30, 2002.

U.S. Department of Education, Office of Special Education Programs, Data Analysis System (DANS).

Annex F: Homeopathic Proving of Mercury

From Allen's *Encyclopedia of Pure Materia Medica*

Mind, easily agitated.

Occasionally his mind seemed to wander.

Frightful images at night.

Hallucinations day and night.

Hallucination of mind, especially at night, with desire to escape.

Delirium; his speech was disconnected, and he would not answer questions; this delirium increased to a violent rage, so that the patient was obliged to be confined in a strait-jacket, with rolling of the eyeballs, clonic spasms, discharge of yellow, frothy liquid from the mouth and nose, and rattling in the trachea, followed by trismus and tetanus.

Delirium.

Delirium, like delirium tremens.

Nightly delirium.

Muttering delirium.

Constant weeping (elder).

Sadness.

Low-spirited.

Spirits depressed.

Anxious.

Attacks of frightful very irritable disposition.

When in the state of tremor, his temper became more irritable, and anger, in turn, so increased the trembling, that he was obliged to sit down to save himself from falling.

Ill-humor.

Ill-humored; the patient was very fretful and peevish; easily excited.

Ill-humor and great irritability.

Fretful mood.

Very fretful mood.

Intellectual.

Slow in answering questions (after thirty-six years).

Thoughts wandering, and impulses whimsical (elder).

Intellect affected; when asked to explain any statement, he becomes confused.

Weakness of intellect and memory.

Intellect very weak; shows every mark of imbecility; smiles foolishly; screams constantly without apparent cause; can speak only a few disconnected words; does not seem to understand the simplest questions, yet appears to know her sister with whom she plays, and repeats a few syllables of what the latter has said to her (younger).

Loss of intellect and memory; a sort of idiocy, which in a few years becomes permanent.

Loss of memory. Complete loss of memory.

Memory slightly affected; forgot the names of persons and places, and was frequently at a loss in endeavoring to recollect the persons to whom he had lent his tools.

Memory weak.

Weakness of memory and loss of will power.

Increasing weakness of memory.

Very poor memory (after thirty-eight years).

Memory very much impaired.

Forgetfulness, with impaired intellect.

Very forgetful.

Loss of consciousness.

Stupor.

Constant disposition to lie down; inclined to sopor, coma.

Delirium; she uncovers herself at night, pulls the straw about, and scolds; during the day she jumps up high both in the open air and in the house (like a wanton, unrestrained person); she talks and scolds a great deal to herself, does not recognize her nearest relatives, spits a great deal and rubs it over the floor with her feet, then partly licks it up; she also frequently licks up cow dung and mud; she puts small stones into her mouth without swallowing them, and complains that they cut her intestines; she passes many clots of blood with the stool; she does violence to no one, but violently resists any one who attempts to touch her; She obeys no one, does not come to her meals, though she usually takes her food and drink irregularly through the day; she looks very pale and haggard, and seems much weaker than before.

He was foolish, played tricks, and made a fool of himself with senseless stuff; in the evening he made a fire in the stove (during the hot summer), laid swords across each other, placed lights in one corner of the room, boots in another, and all the time was fully in earnest; wherewith he was completely indifferent to warmth and cold; but his head was confused and heavy.

He talked senselessly; for example, "see, you have killed a fly on your hand, and just now you forbade me to do it" (which was not so).

He believes that he is losing his reason, thinks that he is dying, with illusions of fantasy; for example sees water running where there is none (in the morning).

He believed that he was enduring infernal torments, without being able to explain himself.

Longing for home.

Was extremely averse to everything, even to music.

Almost involuntary weeping, followed by relief.

While indulging his foolish fancy, he was, however, inclined to weep, and when this paroxysm passed over he was very much exhausted.

Great seriousness, with much indifference, all day; he was very much offended if others laughed over a trifle, and yet was extremely indifferent to everything that took place about him.

Restless, despondent mood; anxiety without particular thoughts.

Much wretchedness and dejection of spirits, with diarrhea.

He wished to die, was averse to everything; indifferent even to the dearest objects.

Anxiety.

Anxiety, which seems as though it would drive him far away, as though he had committed a crime, or as though a misfortune were impending.

Anxiety and apprehension in the blood; did not know what to do; it seemed as though he had committed a crime; without heat; also with a feeling as though he had no control over his senses, all day.

She was constantly anxious and apprehensive; then a sudden affection of the pit of the stomach; her hands began to perspire and her face became hot.

During menstruation, anxiety so that she does not know what to do.

Much anxiety and orgasm of blood, at night, with sticking in the blood vessels.

As soon as she eats, she is attacked with great anxiety, with perspiration on the head and forehead, which seem to her icy cold; she is obliged to go into the open air before the perspiration ceased with want of breath, and sticking in the right side just below the ribs.

Anxiety, as if he had committed a crime.

A feeling as though he had done wrong with loss of ideas.

Very fearful, even to starting up, in the evening.

Extreme fright from slight cause; the whole body trembled; she seemed paralyzed; an excessive glowing heat mounted into the right cheek, which immediately became swollen and bluish-red, and so remained for two hours; she was so effected that she could not again get quiet; all the limbs seemed bruised; violent shaking chills, tottering of the knees, so that she was obliged to lie down.

He had no courage to live.

Was much discontented with himself and his condition, without cause.

Irritability and ill-humor.

Irritable, vexations, active mood.

Ill-humor, associated with anxiety, all day; he constantly thought something disagreeable would happen.

Fretful and peevish all day; he imagined that all his efforts would at last miscarry.

Fretful all day; very much out of sorts and discontented with himself; he had no desire to talk or joke.

Very peevish and intolerant, easily vexed, very suspicious.

Morose all day; extremely taciturn and serious.

Morose and mistrustful all day; he treated his associates almost insultingly, and looked upon everybody as his worst enemy.

Fighting, quarrelsome mood.

Quarrels with everything; would above all have everything right; quarrelsome.

While taking a walk, he has a strong inclination to pinch the noses of the strangers he meets.

Rather indifferent mood.

Extremely indifferent.

Cared for nothing and was indifferent to everything.

He was indifferent to everything in the world; had no desire to eat and yet, when he ate, relished his food and took as much as usual.

Intellectual.

Hurried and rapid talking.

No desire for earnest work.

Talking was irksome; could not read; the head was confused; could work at nothing, and fell asleep while sitting.

Dull and sleepy during the day.

It affects acuteness of thought, makes him dizzy; he does not hear what is spoken, does not comprehend what he is reading, and easily makes mistakes in talking.

Thought is very weak; it is extremely difficult to collect his thoughts, and he makes wrong answers to questions (that he himself notices).

He is unable to calculate; cannot put his mind on anything.

Thoughts entirely vanish.

At times, thought disappears for several minutes.

Distraction of mind; while he was at work at anything, something else constantly came into his mind; thoughts constantly thronged upon each other, from time to time (for several days).

Loss of consciousness and speech; she seems to sleep, but is pulseless, with the usual warmth of the body and with the perfect look of a corpse; after an hour consciousness and some sound of the voice returned; she tried to speak but could not; only after twelve hours did speech return.

He does not know where he is.

Annex G: Resources for Parents on Vaccinations

The following web sites are a good starting point to learn more about the risks of vaccination. These risks are sufficient to demand that all vaccinations be a matter of parental choice, and that each parent be fully informed of the risks. However, the vested political and monetary interests in vaccination, plus the prevailing paradigm that sees them as “good,” will likely continue to work against “truth in advertising” in any government health measures involving vaccination.

Articles

Dispelling Vaccination Myths: An Introduction to the Contradictions Between Medical Science and Immunization Policy
by Alan Phillips, Director Citizens for Healthcare Freedom
http://www.mercola.com/2001/aug/18/vaccine_myths.htm

Vaccination: A Sacrament of Modern Medicine
by Richard Moskowitz, MD
http://www.healthy.net/library/articles/moskowitz/vaccination.htm

Books

Immunization: History, Ethics, Law and Health
by Catherine Diodati M.A.

The Vaccine Guide
by Randall Neustader

Vaccination: 100 Years of Orthodox Research shows that Vaccines Represent a Medical Assault on the Immune System
by Viera Schreibner PhD

Immunization: The Reality Behind the Myth - Second Edition, Revised and Updated
by Walene James

A Shot in the Dark: Why the P in the DPT Vaccination May Be Hazardous to Your Child's Health
by Harris L. Coulter and Barbara Loe Fisher

Vaccination, Social Violence, and Criminality: The Medical Assault on the American Brain
by Harris L. Coulter

How to Raise a Healthy Child in Spite of Your Doctor
by Robert Mendelsohn MD

Vaccination and Immunization
by Leon Chaitow

The Medical Mafia
by Dr. Guyliane Lanctot

And we must remember the impact of vaccines on other family members, and this is an excellent book on the subject:

Vaccine Guide for Dogs and Cats: What Every Pet Lover Should Know
by Catherine J. M. Diodati, M.A.

Video

The University of Calgary's Faculty of Medicine, Department of Physiology and Biophysics: How Mercury Causes Brain Neuron Degeneration

http://commons.ucalgary.ca/mercury/

Web Sites

The links below may come and go over time, but there will always be an up-to-date list on our own website:
www.heilkunst.com/vaccinations

Other websites:

www.vran.org - Vaccination Risk Awareness Network, Canada

www.eaglefoundation.net/Vaccine%20Info.htm - Eagle Foundation

www.whale.to/vaccines.html - Whale Vaccine mega-website

http://chetday.com/novacarticles.html - Medical Journal articles on the dangers of vaccinations

www.vaccines.net - Vaccine Safety Website, USA

http://vaccineinfo.net/index.shtml - Parents Requesting Open Vaccine Education, USA

http://home.san.rr.com/via/ - Vaccine Information & Awareness, USA

www.909shot.com - National Vaccine Information Center, USA

www.geocities.com/Heartland/8148/vac.html#links - Be Informed About Vaccinations, USA

www.vaccinesornot.org - Vaccines or Not?

http://mercola.com/article/vaccines/links.htm - Dr. Mercola's vaccination links and his own vaccination articles

www.nccn.net/~wwithin/vaccine.htm - Informed Parents Vaccination Web page

http://curezone.com/topic/vaccination/ - Cure Zone: Info and articles on the dangers of vaccines

Annex H: Weapons of Mass Destruction

As we were going to print, one of our students sent us this article, which we found so valuable we wanted to include it here, in part:

Inoculations: The True Weapons of Mass Destruction Causing VIDS (Vacine Induced Diseases)

"An Epidemic of Genocide" by Rebecca Carley, M.D. Court Qualified Expert in VIDS and Legal Abuse Syndrome

January 2005

"One basic truth can be used as a foundation for a mountain of lies, and if we dig down deep enough in the mountain of lies, and bring out that truth, to set it on top of the mountain of lies; the entire mountain of lies will crumble under the weight of that one truth. And there is nothing more devastating to a structure of lies than the revelation of the truth upon which the structure of lies was built, because the shock waves of the revelation of the truth reverberate, and continue to reverberate throughout the Earth for generations to follow, awakening even those people who had no desire to be awakened to the truth." (by Delamar Duvaris as written in the preface of "Behold the Pale Horse" by William Gary).

The basic truth that served as the foundation for the mountain of lies known as vaccinations was the observation that mammals which recover from infection with microorganisms acquire natural immunity from further infections. Whenever cytotoxic T cells (the little Pac man cells which devour and neutralize viruses, bacteria, and cancer cells, thus conferring cellular immunity and are also responsible for allograft rejection) and B cells (antibody producing cells which confer humoral immunity by circulating in the body's fluids or "humors", primarily serum or lymph) are activated by various substances foreign to the body called antigens, some of the T and B cells become memory cells. Thus, the next time the individual meets up with that same antigen, the immune system can be quickly triggered to demolish it. This is the process known as natural immunity.

This truth gave birth to a beLIEf that if a foreign antigen was injected into an individual, that individual would then become immune to a future infection. This beLIEf, (you see the lie in the middle), was given the name, "vaccinations". What the promoters of vaccination failed to realize is that secretory IgA (an antibody found predominately in saliva and secretions of the gastrointestinal and respiratory tract mucosa) is the initial normal antibody response to all airborne and ingested pathogens. IgA helps protect against viral infection, agglutinate bacteria, neutralize microbial toxins, and decrease attachment of pathogens to mucosal surfaces. What this author has realized is that bypassing this mucosal aspect of the immune system by directly injecting organisms into the body leads to a corruption in the immune system itself whereby IgA is transmuted into IgE, and/or the B cells are hyperactivated to produce pathologic amounts of self-attacking antibody as well as suppression of cytotoxic T cells (as explained shortly). As a result, the pathogenic viruses or bacteria cannot be eliminated by the immune system and remain in the body, where they cause chronic disease and thus further grow and/or mutate as the individual is exposed to ever more antigens and toxins in the environment. This is especially true with viruses grouped under the term "stealth adapted", which are viruses formed when vaccine viruses combine with viruses from tissues used to culture them, leading to a lack of some critical antigens normally recognized by the cellular immune system. One example is stealth adapted (mutated) cytomegaloviruses which arose from African green monkey (simian) kidney cells when they were used to culture polio virus for live polio virus vaccines. Thus, not only was the vaccinee inoculated with polio, but with the cytomegalovirus as well.

The mechanism by which the immune system is corrupted can best be realized when you understand that the two poles of the immune system (the cellular and humoral mechanisms) have a reciprocal relationship in that when the activity of one pole is increased, the other must decrease. Thus, when one is stimulated, the other is inhibited. Since vaccines activate the B cells to secrete antibody, the cytotoxic (killer) T cells are subsequently suppressed. (In fact, progressive vaccinia (following vaccination with smallpox) occurs in the presence of high titers of circulating antibody to the virus [1] combined with suppressed cytotoxic T cells, leading to spreading of lesions all over the body). This suppression of the cell-mediated response is thus a key factor in the development of cancer and life threatening infections. In fact, the "prevention" of a disease via vaccination is, in reality, an inability to expel organisms due to the suppression of the cell-mediated response. Thus, rather than preventing disease, the disease is actually prevented from ever being resolved. The organisms continue circulating through the body, adapting to the hostile environment by transforming into other organisms depending on acidity, toxicity and other changes to the internal terrain of the body as demonstrated by the works of Professor Antoine Béchamp. He established this prior to the development of the "germ theory" of disease by Louis Pasteur. Pasteur's "germ theory" was a plagiarist's attempt to reshape the truth from Béchamp into his own "original" premise – the beLIEf that germs are out to "attack" us, thereby causing dis-ease. Thus, treatment of infection with antibiotics as well as "prevention" of disease with vaccines are both just corrupted attempts at cutting off the branches of dis-ease, when the root of the cause is a toxic internal environment combined with nutritional deficiency. However, since Pasteur's germ theory was conducive to the profits of the burgeoning pharmaceutical cartels that only manage dis-ease, no mention of the work of Professor Béchamp is made in medical school curricula.

To make matters worse than the suppression of cellular immunity which occurs when vaccines are injected, adjuvants (which are substances added to vaccines to enhance the antibody response) can actually lead to serious side effects themselves. Adjuvants include oil emulsions, mineral compounds (which may contain the toxic metal aluminum), bacterial products, liposomes (which allow delayed release of substances), and squalene. The side effects of adjuvants themselves include hyperactivity of B cells leading to pathologic [2] levels of antibody production, as well as allergic reaction to the adjuvants themselves (as demonstrated in Gulf War I soldiers injected with vaccines containing the adjuvant squalene, to which antibodies were found in many soldiers). Note that the pathologically elevated hyperactivity of antibody production caused by adjuvants also results in a distraction from the other antigens that the immune system encounters "naturally", which must be addressed to maintain health.

In addition to the transmutation of IgA into IgE leading to allergic reactions described shortly, the overall hyperactivity of the humoral (antibody producing) pole of the immune system is, in this author's opinion, the sole cause of all autoimmune diseases. The only thing which determines which autoimmune disease you develop is which tissues in your body are attacked by auto-antibodies [3]. If the inside lining of the gastrointestinal tract (the mucosa) is attacked by auto-antibodies you develop leaky gut syndrome (which leads to food allergies when partially digested food particles are released into the bloodstream, are recognized as antigens foreign to the body, and elicit an antibody response against those food particles that becomes heightened every time that same food is eaten and released into the bloodstream partially digested again). Crohn's disease and colitis are also caused by auto-antibody attack on the mucosa of the GI tract itself. If the islet (insulin producing) cells of the pancreas are attacked by auto-antibodies, you develop insulin dependent (juvenile) diabetes. If the respiratory mucosa is attacked by auto-antibodies, you develop "leaky lung" syndrome where, just as with leaky gut, antigens recognized as foreign to the body which are inhaled are able to traverse the lining of the respiratory tract, causing the creation of antibodies against those antigens (usually dust, mold, pet or pollen antigens). When these substances are inhaled again, IgE (the pathologic form of IgA created after corruption of the immune system due to inoculation rather than inhalation of disease) acts as a reagin [4] and sensitizes mast and basophil cells, causing release of their histamine and slow reacting substance granules on contact with the allergen to produce constriction of the bronchioles leading to asthma. This process is also responsible for the immediate hypersensitivity reaction known as anaphylaxis, which is a potential side effect noted in the Physician's Desk Reference for every vaccine; as well as the wheal and flare reaction of the skin known as hives. If the components of the articular surface of the joints are attacked by auto-antibodies, you develop rheumatoid (or juvenile) arthritis. If the skin is compromised on a chronic basis, you develop "leaky skin" syndrome, where contact antigens which could not otherwise traverse the skin lead to skin allergies to contact antigens (a delayed hypersensitivity reaction where inflammation occurs due to release of soluble factors). Additionally, depending on which level of the skin is attacked by auto-antibodies, (i.e., the epidermis or dermis), you develop eczema, psoriasis or scleroderma. If the kidney tissue is attacked by auto-antibodies, you develop one of the many types of nephritis, depending on which component of renal tissue is attacked (for example, with glomerulonephritis, the basement membrane of the glomerular apparatus within the kidney (which filters blood to form urine) is attacked by auto-antibodies, thus allowing protein to escape from the serum into the urine). If you develop auto-antibodies against thyroid gland tissue, you develop Grave's disease. If you develop auto-antibodies against the tissue of the thymus gland (which is crucial in T cell production and function), you develop myasthenia gravis. If you develop auto-antibodies against the very DNA in the nucleus of all cells, you develop systemic Lupus (thus, the autoimmune potential of DNA vaccines being developed now is self evident; worse yet, DNA components from these vaccines can be incorporated into your DNA, leading to actual genetic changes which could cause extinction of all (vaccinated) life on the Earth, as will be discussed shortly). And on, and on, and on.

The brain and spinal cord can also be attacked with auto-antibodies (which this author refers to as vaccine induced encephalitis), leading to a variety of neurological diseases. The most severe of these, leading to death, are sudden infant death syndrome (SIDS) and most cases of “shaken baby syndrome”. If components of the myelin sheath (the insulating covering of nerve fibers which allows proper nerve conduction) or the actual neurofilaments themselves are attacked by auto-antibodies, the resultant condition is determined solely by the location of the damage done. Such neurological conditions include but are not limited to minimal brain dysfunction, ADD/ADHD, learning disabilities, mental retardation, criminal behavior, the spectrum of pervasive developmental disorders (including autism), multiple sclerosis, Parkinson’s disease, Lou Gehrig’s disease, Guillen (sic) Barre’, seizure disorders, etc., etc. etc. (Please note that other factors are also sometimes involved, such as: the organism which causes Lymes disease, aspartame and mercury in cases of MS; aspartame in seizures; or pesticides in cases of Parkinson’s). Thus, when detoxing to reverse these diseases, these other substances must also be removed to obtain a full recovery. However, the corruption of the immune system caused by the injection of vaccines is a key component in these disease states leading to immune malfunction, and is the reason why an autistic child may also have leaky gut or eczema, etc. Note that myelin production, for the most part, does not begin until after birth. Most myelin is apparently laid down by age 5 years and usually completed by age 10 years, judging by the level of success at various ages in reversing autistic and other neurological VIDS symptoms that this author has observed in hundreds of children by detoxing the viruses with homeopathic nosodes[5], and repairing the immune corruption by simultaneous administration of bovine colostrum (i.e., after 10 years of age, the ability to stop and repair auto-antibody induced damage in the myelin sheath and neurofilaments themselves is dramatically decreased).

In summary, the hyperactivity of the humoral arm of the immune system in autoimmune disease is caused by adjuvants added just for that purpose. However, the damage caused by the autoimmunity itself (i.e., antibody against self) has several mechanisms, including the following:

1. The antigens present in the culture media itself cannot be completely filtered and separated from the organisms cultured thereon. Thus, any antibodies formed against antigens from the culture cells themselves (for example myelin basic protein from chick embryos or the 13 vaccines which now contain aborted human fetal cells) can cross-react to form an autoimmune reaction against the myelin basic protein in your myelin sheath, etc.

2. Molecular mimicry is due to similarity of proteins contained in organisms and mammals. (For example, the measles virus is made up of proteins similar to myelin basic protein; thus, antibodies formed against the measles virus antigens subsequently also cause an auto-antibody attack against myelin basic protein in the myelin sheath due to cross reactivity of these antibodies).

3. Formation of immune complexes occur as antigens and antibodies interlock into clusters which can then become trapped in various tissues, especially the kidneys, lung, skin, joints, or blood vessels. Once trapped, these complexes then set off an inflammatory reaction which lead (sic) to further tissue damage.

4. Intentional inclusion of antigens in vaccines to cause formation of antibodies that attack specific hormones or races (for example, experiments done on women of childbearing age in the Philippines and probably other locations where HCG (human chorionic gonadotropin) [6] placed into vaccines given these women resulted in antibodies against the HCG hormone, and subsequent spontaneous abortion thus occurred when the women became pregnant. It is also this author's hypothesis that the epidemic of vitiligo in people of color (hypo pigmentation of skin caused by auto-antibody attack on melanocytes [7]) is also occurring due to intentional inclusion of melanin in vaccines given to people of color.

Another heinous (and obviously genocidal) creation of the Anti-Hippocratics is the DNA vaccines now being developed. These vaccines contain plasmids, which are closed rings of recombinant DNA that make their way into the nucleus of a cell and instruct the cell to synthesize encoded antigenic proteins [8]. Thus, the very genetic makeup of the individual, plant or animal will be altered to produce a never ending supply of antigens to distract the immune system. These genetic changes will remain as cell division occurs, and will be transmissible to offspring. This is the TRUE "mark of the beast", and could lead to extinction and/or modification (including behavioral) of any group inoculated.

In addition to the above phenomena which lead to simultaneous depression of cellular immune function and hyperactivity of humoral immune function, vaccines also contain other toxic substances which can cause serious side effects themselves. The following ingredients are actually listed on the CDC website with this introductory statement: "Many things in today's world, including food and medicines, have chemicals added to them to prevent the growth of germs and reduce spoilage." Translation: you're already toxic, so what's the big deal with adding more poison? This author's answer to that question is that any immunotoxin can end up being the "straw that breaks the immune system's back" in that individual, leading to dis-ease. This is where genetics is key; i.e., not that what disease you develop is actually caused by some "gene" in most cases; but rather that your genes determine the strength of your immune system (i.e., how many assaults your immune system can take before it reaches critical mass, and you develop a dis-ease).

Some additional ingredients in vaccines (as listed by the CDC on their website) include antibiotics, aluminum gels, formaldehyde, monosodium glutamate (MSG), egg protein, and sulfites. Thus, we have antibiotics (which you could be allergic to); aluminum (which when combined with silicon deficiency, results in the neurofibrillary tangles seen in Alzheimer's disease); formaldehyde (a toxic carcinogenic substance used to preserve dead people); MSG (a potent excitotoxin [9] which, like aspartame, can cause seizures, brain tumors, etc.); egg protein (to which you could have a life threatening anaphylactic reaction); and sulfites (another toxin which we are advised not to consume much of orally, but in vaccines, it is injected directly into the body). Is this not a veritable witch's brew of chemicals, organisms, and animal parts? What the CDC does NOT list is that 13 vaccines at present (and more are in the works) are actually cultured on aborted human fetal tissues (go to www.cogforlife.org for more info). THIS IS CANNIBALISM. Note in this list that they also fail to mention the ethyl-mercury containing preservative thimerosal, which has been the only dangerous substance in vaccines to receive mainstream media attention (albeit most of that being disinformation) after the explosion in the rate of occurrence of autism in the last generation became self-evident proof that vaccines are the causative factor. For, although the scientists working for the medical mafia continue to use statistics to twist and spin their data to make us beLIEve that vaccines are not the cause, too many thousands of parents have watched their children enter the downward spiral into autism after their children received the vaccine which was the straw that broke the back of their child's immune system. No matter what the "white coats" tell these parents, they know the truth!

Mercury (also in dental amalgam fillings) is a highly toxic heavy metal, has been documented to cause cancer, and can be absorbed through the digestive track, skin, and respiratory track. Mercury is 1,000 times more toxic than lead, and is second only to uranium as the most toxic metal. If children receive all recommended vaccines, they will receive many times the "allowable safe limit" for mercury in the first two years of life (as if there is such a thing as a "safe" amount of a toxic poison). Yet, even after Congressional hearings instigated by Congressman Dan Burton (whose own grandchild became autistic after receiving vaccines) resulted in the FDA requesting (not ordering) vaccine manufacturers to remove this toxic heavy metal from their products, mercury is still present in many vaccines.

Although the symptoms of mercury poisoning have been described as identical to the symptoms of autism, it should be noted that most children who descend into the hellish state known as autism do so after the MMR vaccine. The MMR vaccine is one of the few vaccines that do not contain mercury. Thus, it is self-evident that the removal of mercury will not make vaccines "safe". (This is why the mercury is the only thing being addressed at all; because when the people reading this paper realize that the very mechanism by which vaccines corrupt the immune system means that NO vaccine is safe and effective; there will be an evolution of consciousness where the structure of lies telling us vaccines are safe and effective disintegrates.)

The good news is that these VIDS can be reversed using natural remedies (especially homeopathy) contained in the Hippocrates Protocol (www.drcarley.com). This "surgical strike" detoxification approach which has the potential to reverse ALL of the aforementioned conditions under the VIDS umbrella as long as detoxification is started early enough will be the one truth put on top of the mountain of lies (that vaccines are safe and effective) that will cause the entire mountain of vaccine lies to crumble.

This article may be found in full at: http://www.drcarley.com

Annex I: FAQs regarding Heilkunst and Autism

There is no question that we currently face an unprecedented tragedy in the form of a profound disturbance in the health of our children at all levels - body, mind, soul and spirit. We are all witnesses to a plague of autism, as the usual alphabet soup of behavioral disorders - ADHD, ADD, ODD, PDD etc.

While the statisticians and the supposed experts continue to argue over cause and effect, and search for incontrovertible "proof," with research mainly carried out within a limited, and largely outmoded, bio-chemical paradigm, the tragedy continues to strike individuals and their families by the thousands, with little real relief and only vague hopes in continued research. But research that does not address the many *true* causes of autism and other behavioral conditions has little chance of doing anything other than palliating the symptoms.

QUESTION: Do you think autism is an actual disease?

> **ANSWER:** Autism, ADD, ADHD, PDD and ODD are not diseases in our assessment, but only labels placed on observed behavior that is not considered natural or that is disruptive to the child or to others. We could say that they are disease conditions.
>
> To the extent that the label is correct (and this is often not the case with ADD, ADHD for example) the causes still remain hidden, speculative and confusing. No two cases are the same in all, or even in many, respects. The causes remain hidden because the diagnosis is effectively an illusion. The disorder or condition is real, but it is only the result of something deeper that is not identified. To give something a name does not make it a disease.

A true diagnosis always contains the remedy within it. For example, a diagnosis of a lack of vitamin C, where this is truly the case, tells you exactly what you must do for the cure – provide vitamin C. But if the cause is not a lack of vitamin C, then extra vitamin C may *help* the symptoms, but it will *not* remove the underlying cause. And these deeper causes can be one or more of a long list of shocks or stresses to the system.

QUESTION: Do you see autism as a behavioral problem?

ANSWER: Autism and the other disorders mentioned produce disturbed behavior, but in our experience and understanding they are not a behavioral problem. They are instead the product of actual traumas to the system, which place it in shock, weakening the immune system and calling forth a response from the organism to defend itself (this produces most of the symptoms we notice). This is much like a shell-shocked soldier coming back from war.

The list of potential and actual shocks to the system is virtually endless, particularly if we include the host of interventions by the modern medical system (some necessary and even life-saving in extreme cases, but shocks to the system nonetheless).

These fall into one or the other of the following categories:

- Inherited weaknesses in terms of the (ill) health of the parents and earlier generations. Children can only be as healthy as the parents and, if untreated, the miasms manifest symptoms earlier and earlier and more and more insidiously in each new generation
- Stresses and traumas during pregnancy (ultrasounds, amniocentesis, drugs, antibiotics, poor diet, emotional stresses, accidents)
- Birth interventions (induction, epidural, episiotomy, forceps, suctioning, drugs, C-section)
- Vaccinations, particularly the ones within the first few months and years of life, and notably shortly after birth, such as the Hepatitis

B or anti-Tubercular vaccines. Most children today have had more than 30 shots by the time they are three years old. (For more information on resources on the negative effects of vaccinations, see our links page.)

- Accidents (broken bones, concussions, spinal injuries, deep wounds, animal bites, etc.)
- Emotional shocks (deaths, frights, fears, suppressed emotions, etc.) of any sort - it is the *reaction* of the person rather than the actual shock itself that is more of a determinant
- Iatrogenic diseases - drugs, antibiotics, surgeries
- Poor diet and exposure to various chemicals
- Inherited diseases that affect how the genetic code functions

QUESTION: Is autism caused by toxic metals, such as mercury in vaccines, or by a disorder in gut flora and fauna, or maybe a poor diet?

ANSWER: It is true that toxic metals and the other factors mentioned can contribute to the emergence of an autistic condition and other behavioral problems. In some cases one of the other factors, or a combination of such factors, may play a large role. In those cases addressing the factors through detoxification and dietary approaches may help considerably. However, in many other cases such efforts have little or no positive effect although they are still good for overall health, and they may require a great deal of effort, time, money and discipline.

Finally, though heroic measures in diet and detoxification can certainly help improve behavior and health, they do not usually get at the underlying *causes* and must be followed up with, or done parallel to, a treatment that *is* able to remove these causes.

QUESTION: Why do most autistic children have high doses of heavy metals?

ANSWER: There can be some logical reasons, such as the high number of vaccines with mercury (thimerosal) and other metal products. There is no question that the *true* safe levels of exposure for these heavy metals is zero, and that this is not the case in our world.

However, we are all exposed to heavy metals, but not all of us seem to hold them or carry them around in our systems. The deeper problem lies in the fact that autistic children hang on to these metals rather than allowing their natural detoxification system to neutralize and remove them. Why?

Our research strongly suggests that it's because of the traumas to their system and inherited weaknesses that create a form of "armoring" at the cellular level that mirrors that of the level of the psyche. Once these traumas are removed, the cells then allow the toxins to leave and be processed by the normal detoxification system of the body.

Although it may seem strange, our cases point to the possibility that the body itself, under certain situations of stress, will produce some if not all of the heavy metals. In the more traditional medical system of the past, the various metals were seen to have a relationship to certain disease states and to possess healing qualities.

Thus, as is the case with many viruses, the heavy metals may be as much the *result*, as the cause, of the disease condition. This is also strongly suggested by the fact that in many cases the heavy metal levels cannot be accounted for by environmental exposure alone, and that not all persons in the identical environment carry the same level of heavy metals, and indeed, other toxins.

QUESTION: Why is it that what works for one child doesn't work for mine?

ANSWER: The label a child is given is not a true diagnosis, but more of a description. We say it is descriptive, not disclosive, of the cause as a true diagnosis must be. Thus, the label "Autism" hides the many and varying factors in each case that are responsible for the disorder termed autism, or ADD or ADHD, etc. Your child is unique in the combination and sequence of events that led to his or her autistic condition, and in the family history. The challenge is to find this combination and sequence for each individual and to treat for it correctly.

QUESTION: How can homeopathy and Heilkunst help my child?

ANSWER: Heilkunst is an approach to treatment that combines the best of regimenal measures (diet, detoxification, etc.) and medicine, all based on the principles of natural law. While any substance can be used to have an *effect* (usually to remove a symptom), this does not mean that it is being used properly, that is, according to the laws that nature has set down.

We all are products of nature and any treatment must ultimately follow natural law principles. If not, it is acting only palliatively (temporary relief) or worse, suppressively. If the symptoms are suppressed, the cause of the problem is *not* removed and the symptoms may return or the cause goes underground where it will cause other problems later in time.

The core of Heilkunst is an approach to identifying and then removing the underlying causes of autism and other behavioral conditions using a rational, natural and systematic, sequential treatment. The use of medicines that are non-toxic, non-invasive and curative of the underlying shocks gives it a high degree of success.

While each case is unique, we have been able to help achieve significant improvement, including removal of the autistic and other behavioral conditions, in cases where nothing else seemed to be working.

QUESTION: How long does the treatment take?

ANSWER: Treatment will vary from case to case, but generally takes about one or two years to complete to the first level (which is usually sufficient for significant improvement). Improvement will often be noticed in the first three to six months, but it takes longer to get deeper improvement and to make it more permanent. In difficult cases, we may require longer treatment to get at the deeper root causes, and even here the results are very promising.

QUESTION: Is the improvement permanent?

ANSWER: Since we are removing the underlying *causes* of the condition, to the extent that it is curable, the condition is permanently removed. While a child may take his or her constitutional remedy occasionally to maintain good health under the stresses of life, or an occasional remedy for first aid or acute complaints, there is no need to continue taking remedies beyond the treatment period.

QUESTION: Why is this approach not better known?

ANSWER: The approach we use is based on a long tradition of homeopathic medical practice, which is the second most popular system of medicine in the world. It is less-well known in North America because of the greater dominance of the drug companies both in terms of medical training and adverti$ing. The use of bio-energetic medicines on the basis of natural law principles also goes against the current bio-chemical paradigm that dominates Western medicine.

QUESTION: What is the difference between Heilkunst and homeopathy?

ANSWER: Heilkunst is the term given to the *complete* medical system discovered and developed by Dr. Samuel Hahnemann more than 200 years ago. Dr. Hahnemann is also known as the founder of homeopathy, however this is only *one part* of his complete medical system. And while homeopathy can be effective in some cases, it is not as effective as consistently as Hahnemann's complete approach, particularly in complex, chronic cases.

QUESTION: Is there evidence of the effectiveness of homeopathy?

ANSWER: While most modern research is conducted by drug companies on patentable drugs, there is a long history of recorded clinical success with homeopathic medicines, as well as some clinical trials using modern methods (see www.homeopathic.com/articles/research/index.php).

Polymorphism?

Diagnosis

THRO KNOWING.

Dynamis < generative. / sustentive.

Health care vs. Disease management

Thomas Kuhn - prevailing paradigm limits thinking.

"Poor diet AND nutrition"?